theclinics.com

INFECTIOUS DISEASE CLINICS OF NORTH AMERICA

Hepatitis

CONSULTING EDITOR
Robert C. Moellering, Jr, MD

March 2006 • Volume 20 • Number 1

SAUNDERS
An Imprint of Elsevier, Inc.
PHILADELPHIA LONDON TORONTO MONTREAL SYDNEY TOKYO

W.B. SAUNDERS COMPANY
A Division of Elsevier Inc.

Elsevier, Inc., 1600 John F. Kennedy Blvd., Suite 1800, Philadelphia, PA 19103-2899.

http://www.theclinics.com

INFECTIOUS DISEASE CLINICS OF NORTH AMERICA
March 2006
Editor: Rachel Glover

Volume 20, Number 1
ISSN 0891–5520
ISBN 1-4160-3732-2

Infectious Disease Clinics of North America (ISSN 0891–5520) is published in March, June, September, and December (For Post Office use only: volume 20 issue 1 of 4) by W.B. Saunders, 360 Park Avenue South, New York, NY 10010-1710. Business and Editorial Offices: 1600 John F. Kennedy Blvd., Suite 1800, Philadelphia, PA 19103-2899. Accounting and Circulation Offices: 6277 Sea Harbor Drive, Orlando, FL 32887-4800. Periodicals postage paid at New York, NY and additional mailing offices. Subscription prices are $170.00 per year for US individuals, $285.00 per year for US institutions, $85.00 per year for US students, $200.00 per year for Canadian individuals, $345.00 per year for Canadian institutions, $225.00 per year for international individuals, $345.00 per year for international institutions, and $110.00 per year for Canadian and foreign students. To receive student rate, orders must be accompained by name of affiliated institution, date of term, and the *signature* of program/residency coordinator on institution letterhead. Orders will be billed at individual rate until proof of status is received. Foreign air speed delivery is included in all *Clinics* subscription prices. All prices are subject to change without notice. **POSTMASTER**: Send address changes to *Infectious Disease Clinics of North America*, Elsevier Periodicals Customer Service, 6277 Sea Harbor Drive, Orlando, FL 32887-4800. **Customer Service: 1-800-654-2452 (US). From outside of the US, call 1-407-345-4000. E-mail: hhspcs@wbsaunders.com**.

Infectious Disease Clinics of North America is also published in Spanish by Editorial Inter-Médica, Junin 917, 1er A 1113, Buenos Aires, Argentina.

Reprints. For copies of 100 or more, of articles in this publication, please contact the Commercial Reprints Department, Elsevier Inc., 360 Park Avenue South, New York, New York 10010-1710. Tel. (212) 633-3813, Fax: (212) 462-1935, email: reprints@elsevier.com.

Infectious Disease Clinics of North America is covered in *Index Medicus, Current Contents/Clinical Medicine, Science Citation Alert, SCISEARCH, and Research Alert.*

Printed in the United States of America.

CONSULTING EDITOR

ROBERT C. MOELLERING, Jr, MD, Herrman L. Blumgart Professor of Medical Research, Harvard Medical School; and Physician-in-Chief and Chairman, Department of Medicine, Beth Israel Deaconess Medical Center, Boston, Massachusetts

CONTRIBUTORS

NEZAM H. AFDHAL, MD, Department of Medicine, Harvard Medical School; The Liver Center, Beth Israel Deaconess Medical Center, Boston, Massachusetts

FURQAAN AHMED, MD, Division of Hepatology and Gastroenterology, Weill Medical College of Cornell University, New York, New York

SCOTT W. BIGGINS, MD, Division of Gastroenterology, Department of Medicine, University of California, San Francisco, San Francisco, California

RAMSEY C. CHEUNG, MD, Department of Hepatology, VA Palo Alto Health Care System; Division of Gastroenterology and Hepatology, Stanford University School of Medicine, Palo Alto, California

ADRIAN M. DI BISCEGLIE, MD, Division of Gastroenterology and Hepatology, Department of Internal Medicine, Saint Louis University Liver Center, St. Louis, Missouri

EDWARD C. DOO, MD, Liver Disease Research Branch, National Institute of Diabetes and Digestive and Kidney Diseases, National Institutes of Health, Bethesda, Maryland

LAWRENCE S. FRIEDMAN, MD, Department of Medicine, Harvard Medical School, Boston; Department of Medicine, Newton-Wellesley Hospital, Newton; Department of Medicine, Massachusetts General Hospital, Boston, Massachusetts

MARC G. GHANY, MD, Liver Diseases Section, National Institute of Diabetes and Digestive and Kidney Diseases, National Institutes of Health, Bethesda, Maryland

JEFFREY S. GLENN, MD, PhD, Division of Gastroenterology and Hepatology, Stanford University School of Medicine and Palo Alto Veterans Administration Medical Center, Palo Alto, California

PAUL H. HAYASHI, MD, Division of Gastroenterology and Hepatology, Department of Internal Medicine, Saint Louis University Liver Center, St. Louis, Missouri

IRA M. JACOBSON, MD, Division of Hepatology and Gastroenterology, Weill Medical College of Cornell University, New York, New York

EMMET B. KEEFFE, MD, Division of Gastroenterology and Hepatology, Stanford University School of Medicine, Palo Alto, California

SANGIK OH, MD, MMSc, Department of Medicine, Harvard Medical School; The Liver Center, Beth Israel Deaconess Medical Center, Boston, Massachusetts

JULIE C. SERVOSS, MD, Department of Medicine, Harvard Medical School; Gastrointestinal Unit, Massachusetts General Hospital, Boston, Massachusetts

AMRITA SETHI, MD, Hepatology Section, Virginia Commonwealth University Medical Center, Richmond, Virginia

MITCHELL L. SHIFFMAN, MD, Hepatology Section, Virginia Commonwealth University Medical Center, Richmond, Virginia

NORAH A. TERRAULT, MD, MPH, Division of Gastroenterology, Department of Medicine, University of California, San Francisco, San Francisco, California

ANDY S. YU, MD, Pacific Gastroenterology, San Jose, California

CONTENTS

Preface **xi**
Robert C. Moellering, Jr

The Progression of Hepatitis B– and C–Infections to Chronic Liver Disease and Hepatocellular Carcinoma: Presentation, Diagnosis, Screening, Prevention, and Treatment of Hepatocellular Carcinoma **1**
Paul H. Hayashi and Adrian M. Di Bisceglie

Patients with or at risk for hepatocellular carcinoma (HCC) present special challenges to the clinician. Despite improving understanding of HCC, current guidelines and treatment algorithms are still inadequate. Team coordination and expertise are highly important. In this article, some of the challenging and controversial issues regarding HCC detection, diagnosis, prevention, and care are reviewed, with particular emphasis on hepatitis B– and C–associated HCC. Although not always evidenced-based, practice guidelines or standard of care practices are summarized.

Hepatitis B Vaccines **27**
Andy S. Yu, Ramsey C. Cheung, and Emmet B. Keeffe

Immunization is the most effective way to prevent transmission of hepatitis B virus (HBV) and the development of acute or chronic hepatitis B. The strategy to eliminate HBV transmission in the United States is to vaccinate all newborn infants, children, and adolescents, as well as high-risk adults. Postexposure prophylaxis is advocated after a documented exposure, depending on vaccination history and antibody to hepatitis B surface antigen (anti–HBs) status. Seroprotection after hepatitis B vaccination, defined as anti–HBs ε 10 mIU/mL, is achieved in more than 95% of subjects. Hepatitis B vaccines are very well tolerated with usually minimal adverse effects. Increasing age, male gender, obesity, tobacco smoking, and immunocompromising chronic diseases are predictors of nonresponse to vaccination.

Serologic and Molecular Diagnosis of Hepatitis B Virus 47
Julie C. Servoss and Lawrence S. Friedman

Since the discovery in the 1960s of "Australia antigen," subsequently determined to be hepatitis B surface antigen, serologic assays for hepatitis B virus (HBV) have expanded and evolved. More recently, molecular biology-based techniques have allowed the detection and quantification of HBV DNA in serum. In the past decade, improvements in the sensitivity of these molecular assays have allowed the detection of as few as 10 copies of HBV DNA per milliliter of serum. The combined use of serologic and molecular assays for the diagnosis of HBV infection has resulted in more precise definitions of chronic HBV infection. Molecular assays have become essential to defining responses to antiviral treatment.

Assessment and Management of Chronic Hepatitis B 63
Marc G. Ghany and Edward C. Doo

Chronic hepatitis B (CHB) is a major worldwide cause of chronic liver disease and a significant public health issue. Three predominant clinical presentations are recognized: hepatitis B e antigen (HBeAg) or typical CHB, HBeAg-negative or atypical CHB, and inactive CHB. The natural history of CHB infection in an individual may be dominated by one or a combination of these clinical presentations in a sequential fashion. These variations in clinical presentations reflect the viral-host immunology dynamics that form the basis for the development of liver disease. Therapy has been problematic in the past. There are three licensed drugs available for therapy of CHB with varied mechanisms of action. This has introduced the concept of tailored therapy for the individual patient. Many promising new agents and therapeutic approaches should become available in the near future.

Molecular Virology of the Hepatitis C Virus: Implication for Novel Therapies 81
Jeffrey S. Glenn

The study of hepatitis C virus (HCV) molecular virology is helping to shape the future of our anti-HCV strategies by identifying new antiviral targets. With the advent of agents that specifically target individual HCV proteins, HCV-specific therapy has arrived. Key to these efforts is the development of high-efficiency HCV replicons. The future effective pharmacologic control of HCV will likely consist of a cocktail of simultaneously administered virus-specific agents with independent targets, which should minimize the emergence of resistance against any single agent. The way we treat HCV should change dramatically over the next few years.

Antiviral Therapy for Treatment Naïve Patients with Hepatitis C Virus 99
Sangik Oh and Nezam H. Afdhal

This article focuses on the most recent therapies for patients with hepatitis C virus (HCV) who are naïve to therapy. The primary end point for the treatment of naïve HCV patients is viral eradication or a sustained virological response, which is defined as the absence of HCV in the serum, as detected by a sensitive polymerase chain reaction test, 24 weeks after stopping antiviral therapy. Recent data suggest that an SVR can be equated with a biochemical, virological, and histological response that is sustained for up to 5 years and is conceptually a cure of HCV in 90% of patients.

Approach to the Management of Patients with Chronic Hepatitis C Who Failed to Achieve Sustained Virologic Response **115**
Amrita Sethi and Mitchell L. Shiffman

The combination of peginterferon and ribavirin is the most effective therapy for patients with chronic hepatitis C virus (HCV) infection. Although more than half of all patients are able to achieve a sustained virologic response (SVR), a significant proportion of patients, particularly those with genotype 1, fail to have undetectable HCV RNA during treatment or relapse after completing therapy with return of detectable HCV RNA. The management of these patients creates a formidable challenge. This article outlines various strategies for patients who have failed to achieve SVR and discusses the merits of different approaches to management.

Treatment of Relapsers After Combination Therapy for Chronic Hepatitis C **137**
Furqaan Ahmed and Ira M. Jacobson

A significant number of patients with chronic hepatitis C (CHC) relapse after treatment. As therapy for CHC has improved over the last decade, the issue of retreating patients who did not achieve a sustained virologic response (SVR) with previous treatment regimens frequently arises. Several studies have assessed the efficacy of retreating patients who have previously relapsed to standard interferon monotherapy or standard interferon and ribavirin combination therapy. Patients who have relapsed after therapy have significantly higher SVR rates than those who are nonresponders to therapy and should be considered candidates for retreatment. Predictors of a favorable response to therapy in naïve patients appear to also predict response to therapy in patients who have relapsed previously.

Management of Recurrent Hepatitis C in Liver Transplant Recipients **155**
Scott W. Biggins and Norah A. Terrault

Chronic hepatitis C virus (HCV) infection is the most common indication for liver transplantation in the United States and Europe, and more than 20,000 patients worldwide have undergone transplantation for complications of chronic hepatitis C. In North America, HCV accounts for 15% to 50% of the liver transplants performed

in United States transplant programs. To maximize the long-term survival of liver transplant recipients who have HCV infection, eradication of infection is the ultimate goal. Pretransplant antiviral therapy with the goal of achieving viral eradication before transplantation is a consideration in some patients, especially those who have mildly decompensated liver disease. This article focuses on the management of liver transplant recipients who have HCV infection at the time of transplantation. Prophylactic and preemptive therapies, as well as treatment of established recurrent disease, are the strategies reviewed.

Index **175**

FORTHCOMING ISSUES

June 2006

Bioterrorism
Nancy Khardori, MD, *Guest Editor*

September 2006

Fungal Infections
Thomas F. Patterson, MD, FACP
Guest Editor

RECENT ISSUES

December 2005

Update on Musculoskeletal Infections
John J. Ross, MD, *Guest Editor*

September 2005

Pediatric Infectious Disease
Jeffrey L. Blumer, MD, PhD, and
Philip Toltzis, MD, *Guest Editors*

June 2005

Sexually Transmitted Infections
Jonathan M. Zenilman, MD, *Guest Editor*

ELSEVIER
SAUNDERS

Infect Dis Clin N Am
20 (2006) xi–xii

INFECTIOUS
DISEASE CLINICS
OF NORTH AMERICA

Preface

Hepatitis

Several viruses are capable of causing hepatic inflammation. These include the Epstein-Barr virus, cytomegalovirus, herpes simplex virus, mumps, rubella, rubeola and varicella-zoster viruses, yellow fever virus, Coxsackie viruses, and adenoviruses. In most cases, infection or inflammation of the liver is part of a systemic infection with the above agents. In addition, there are a number of viruses that are primarily hepatotropic and are given alphabetical designations: hepatitis A–E. Several other viruses that were initially thought to cause posttransfusion hepatitis, including hepatitis G virus or GBV-C and SEN viruses, are not currently believed to be human pathogens. Of the truly hepatotropic viruses, hepatitis A and hepatitis E generally produce self-limited disease, although fulminant hepatic failure has been reported in up to 1%–2% of infected individuals. Hepatitis D virus (or the delta agent) can produce coinfections in patients who are infected with hepatitis B, but it appears to be incapable of causing serious disease in the absence of hepatitis B virus. Hepatitis B and C viruses are arguably the most important viruses of this group. In addition to acute infections, exposure to these viruses frequently results in a chronic persistent infection that may remain asymptomatic or lead to cirrhosis, liver failure, and hepatocellular carcinoma. Chronic infections with hepatitis C virus are currently responsible for an increasing percentage of liver transplantations performed in the United States and elsewhere. Because of the large number of patients worldwide who suffer from chronic infections with these two agents, they are arguably the most important viral cause of carcinoma in the world. In recent years, we have learned a great deal about the biology of hepatitis B and C viruses and have gained increasing knowledge of the pathophysiology of the disease they cause in the liver. Concomitant with our understanding of these processes has been the development of a variety of therapeutic modalities, ranging from relatively specific, classic antiviral agents (including lamivudine, adefovir, tenofovir, ribavirin, and a number of new investigational agents) to drugs such as interferon-α, which also have immunomodulatory effects. Vaccine strategies likewise play an important role in preventing hepatitis B. The rapidity of new developments in our understanding of the pathophysiology and management of infections due to hepatitis B and C

0891-5520/06/$ - see front matter
doi:10.1016/j.idc.2006.01.008

make it increasingly difficult for the practicing physician to keep up with the field.

For these reasons, we have assembled in this issue of the *Infectious Disease Clinics of North America* a series of articles written by experts in the field of hepatitis B and C infections. Taken in aggregate, they provide useful, lucid, up-to-date information on the management of hepatitis B and C infections.

Robert C. Moellering, Jr, MD
Harvard Medical School
Department of Medicine
Beth Israel Deaconess Medical Center
110 Francis Street, Suite 6A
Boston, MA 02215, USA

E-mail address: rmoeller@bidmc.harvard.edu

ELSEVIER
SAUNDERS

Infect Dis Clin N Am
20 (2006) 1–25

INFECTIOUS
DISEASE CLINICS
OF NORTH AMERICA

The Progression of Hepatitis B– and C–Infections to Chronic Liver Disease and Hepatocellular Carcinoma: Presentation, Diagnosis, Screening, Prevention, and Treatment of Hepatocellular Carcinoma

Paul H. Hayashi, MD*, Adrian M. Di Bisceglie, MD

Division of Gastroenterology and Hepatology, Department of Internal Medicine, Saint Louis University Liver Center, 3635 Vista Avenue, St. Louis, MO 63110–0250, USA

Patients with, or at risk for, hepatocellular carcinoma (HCC) present special challenges to the clinician. Despite improved understanding of HCC, current guidelines and treatment algorithms are still inadequate. The gastroenterologist or primary care physician may provide screening and prevention, but clinical care after HCC has occurred is a specialized task. A multidisciplinary team including a hepatologist, oncologist, transplant surgeon, interventional radiologist, and liver histopathologist may be needed. Team coordination and expertise is highly important, and most available at tertiary care referral centers. In this article, some of the challenging and controversial issues regarding HCC detection, diagnosis, prevention, and care are reviewed, with particular emphasis on hepatitis B– and C–associated HCC. Although not always evidenced-based, practice guidelines or standard of care practices are summarized.

Clinical presentation

The clinical presentation of HCC ranges from catastrophic tumor rupture into the peritoneum to incidental cancer diagnosed by abdominal imaging.

A version of this article originally appeared in the 89:2 issue of The Medical Clinics of North America.

* Corresponding author.

E-mail address: hayaship@slu.edu (P.H. Hayashi).

doi:10.1016/j.idc.2006.01.003

The most common symptoms are abdominal pain (often right upper quadrant) and weight loss. These symptoms may be more common in areas of endemic chronic hepatitis B and high incidence of HCC [1]. HCC may also lead to hepatic insufficiency by displacement of noncancerous hepatocytes. Cancer extension into the portal vein or its branches may lead to thrombosis and increased portal hypertension. HCC should be suspected in any cirrhotic patient presenting with worsening hepatic function manifested by increased jaundice, encephalopathy, or portal hypertension (ie, ascites, variceal bleeding).

Catastrophic bleeding from tumor rupture is rare. It usually arises from an HCC lesion near the hepatic surface that has outgrown its blood supply [2]. Paraneoplastic symptoms, such as diarrhea, polycythemia, hypercalcemia, hypoglycemia, and feminization, rarely occur. These cases presumably arise from hormones produced by tumor cells. HCC can rarely grow into the hepatic veins and right atrium producing cardiac symptoms [3].

Typical findings on physical examination include cachexia, hepatomegaly, and a firm hepatic edge. Signs of cirrhosis, such as clubbing, palmer erythema, jaundice, and ascites, may occur. Because the blood supply to HCC is arterial, a bruit may be auscultated over the liver. When the tumor involves the liver capsule, a rub may be auscultated during inhalation and exhalation. The rub is often low pitched and sounds like a rumble in contrast to the higher pitched pericardial rub.

Diagnosis

HCC in cirrhotic patients is diagnosed by (1) alpha fetoprotein (AFP) level, (2) imaging studies, and (3) histologic diagnosis. The AFP level is normally less than 15 to 20 ng/mL in adults. The higher the AFP level, the more specific it is for HCC. An AFP greater than 400 ng/mL in a cirrhotic with a vascular hepatic mass on imaging is diagnostic. Unfortunately, many HCC cases have only modestly elevated AFP values. Sensitivities are as low as 45% even for a low cutoff of 20 ng/mL [4]. Moreover, hepatocyte regeneration during and after flares in chronic hepatitis may increase AFP levels in the absence of HCC. Other serologic markers, such as des γ-carboxyprothrombin and glypican-3, have shown promise but are not widely used clinically in the United States [5,6].

Imaging studies, including abdominal ultrasound (US), contrast-enhanced CT, and MRI, are useful. The latter two modalities rely on characteristic vascular qualities to identify lesions. Virtually all HCCs are perfused by the hepatic artery rather than the portal venous system. Large HCCs are usually easy to identify, but small lesions (<2–3 cm) may have subtle vascular markings. CT and MRI scans must include images taken before, during, and after contrast administration (multiphased). An experienced body-imaging radiologist is invaluable in interpreting these tests. Indeed, the choice of CT or MRI for HCC diagnosis often depends on center expertise and preference. US is also quite useful, but a lesion detected on US generally requires an MRI or CT for better characterization. Nevertheless, positive predictive values for CT and MRI can be as low as 37% to 69%, particularly for lesions less than 1 to 2 cm [7,8]. Sonographic contrast materials can be injected into a peripheral vein and cross pulmonary microvasculature to produce air bubbles in the hepatic artery. This diagnostic technique is currently experimental [9,10]. Finally, invasive imaging studies, such as hepatic artery angiogram, and CT and MRI angiography, may increase accuracy [11,12] but are not widely used.

Some experts recommend needle biopsy under imaging guidance partly because lymphoma and nonmalignant lesions can masquerade as HCC [13]. Tissue diagnosis, however, is neither always necessary nor feasible. Biopsies entail some risk. Patients with HCC often have end-stage cirrhosis with coagulopathy, thrombocytopenia, or ascites, all of which increase the risk of bleeding. Small tumors may be difficult to reach by percutaneous biopsy. Cancer cells can rarely seed along the biopsy needle track. Earlier large studies reported a risk of about 0.003% to 0.009% of seeding [14], but more recent studies report a 1% to 2% risk [15,16]. In some studies, the false-negative rate of biopsies is as high as 10% to 40%, particularly for small tumors, because of inadequate samples or sampling error [15,16]. The histopathologic criterion separating dysplastic regenerative nodules from malignancy can be ambiguous. Repeat biopsy does not significantly decrease the false-negative rate [13,16].

Generally accepted guidelines provide criteria for HCC, as published by the European Association for the Study of Liver Disease in 2001 (Box 1) [17]. Note that criteria 2 and 3 apply only in the setting of cirrhosis. The United Network for Organ Sharing (UNOS) in the United States has similar guidelines as described later in the liver transplantation section.

Screening

Screening for HCC remains controversial. HCC meets several criteria for cost-effective screening, including an identifiable risk group (cirrhotic

Box 1. European Association for the Study of Liver Disease hepatocellular carcinoma diagnostic criteria

1. Cytohistopathologic diagnosis or
2. >2-cm arterial hypervascular lesion detected by two coincident imaging techniques in the setting of cirrhosis or
3. >2-cm arterial hypervascular lesion detected by one imaging technique with serum AFP >400 ng/mL in the setting of cirrhosis

patients), a long latent phase, widely available screening tests (US and serum AFP), and potentially curative treatment for early disease (resection, transplantation). These very characteristics, however, have made it difficult to perform a randomized, controlled study. Few patients or institutional review boards accept a study in which controls do not undergo screening until a proportion presents with symptomatic HCC. Patients with symptomatic HCC typically have advanced disease and a poor prognosis. Although screening for HCC makes intuitive sense, questions regarding inadequate sensitivity, specificity, and positive predictive values of screening tests and cost-effectiveness continue to be raised. No medical organization or association has promulgated clear screening guidelines.

Inaccuracies in imaging and AFP interpretation raise concerns about screening. Screening effectiveness depends greatly on the sensitivity and negative predictive value of the tests. Cost effectiveness also depends on the specificity and positive predictive value because chasing false-positive results incurs costs and potential morbidity. The currently available imaging modalities (eg, US or CT) and the serum AFP levels are inadequately sensitive. US, CT, and MRI sensitivities are fine for large lesions (75%–89%), but poor for small lesions (28%–43%) [18]. Because screening is most needed to detect early, small tumors, US, CT, and MRI are inadequate screening tools [4]. The AFP is considered a moderately sensitive test, with a 45% to 100% sensitivity at cutoffs of 10 to 19 ng/mL. Moreover, specificity remains a problem at 70% [4].

Positive predictive value is highly pertinent to clinicians. For example, even if an AFP test has a specificity and sensitivity of 90%, the positive predictive value is only 50% in a population of cirrhotics with a 10% prevalence of HCC (Fig. 1). A test with excellent sensitivity and specificity may be reduced to a coin flip in clinical practice. Some have argued for the abandonment of AFP screening based on this clinical problem [19]. Imaging studies have similar problems. Lack of clearly effective screening tools and good outcomes data results in cost estimates ranging widely from a reasonable $35,000 to a prohibitive $284,000 per year of life saved by screening regimens [20,21].

Nevertheless, the evidence for screening is compelling. Cohort and case-control studies show that patients with HCC detected by screening have significantly earlier cancers at diagnosis, are more likely to undergo curative therapy, and have increased survival time. McMahon et al [22] prospectively analyzed their 16-year experience with twice annual screening of HBsAg-positive Alaska natives using serum AFP. They detected 32 patients with HCC in about 26,000 AFP tests. All but one had tumors less than 6 cm, and 22 patients underwent attempted curative resection. Survival at 5 and 10 years from diagnosis was significantly better than in historical controls not enrolled in a screening program. In a retrospective cohort study of 308 patients with HCC from Hong Kong [23], the 142 patients who were diagnosed through screening with AFP or US had significantly smaller tumors than the patients presenting with symptoms (3.5 cm versus 8.1 cm,

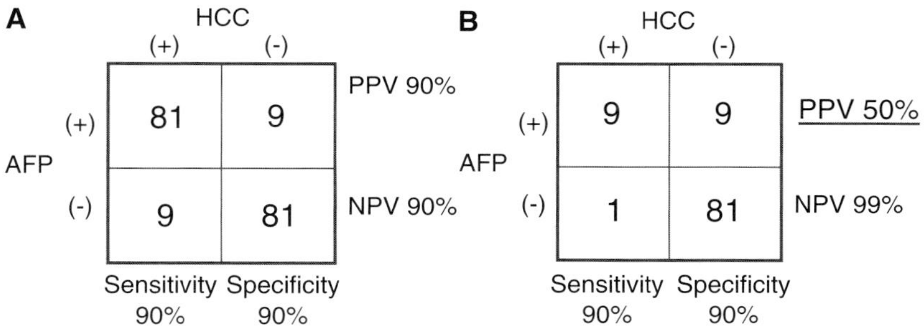

A
HCC
(+)
(-)
AFP
(+)
(-)
81
9
9
81
PPV 90%
NPV 90%
Sensitivity 90%
Specificity 90%
B
HCC
(+)
(-)
AFP
(+)
(-)
9
9
1
81
PPV 50%
NPV 99%
Sensitivity 90%
Specificity 90%

Fig. 1. Hypothetical example demonstrating a problem with using the serum AFP level as a screening test for HCC. (*A*) Promising sensitivity and specificity in a cohort study translates into (*B*) a low positive predictive value in the clinical setting when the prevalence of HCC is only 10%. AFP, alpha fetoprotein; NPV, negative predictive value; PPV, positive predictive value.

$P < .0001$). Resectability and survival were also significantly better in those diagnosed through screening. In a study of 32 patients diagnosed with HCC by screening with US and AFP among 602 patients with chronic viral hepatitis in Los Angeles [24], 18 had single, small tumors possibly amenable to curative treatment. These studies are, however, subject to lead-time and selection biases.

The recent change in priority of patients with HCC for liver transplantation provides another argument for screening. In 2002, the Model for End-stage Liver Disease (MELD) score became the basis for prioritizing patients. In this scoring system, patients with HCC were assigned higher scores and the rate of transplantation for these patients tripled in the first year [25]. Liver transplantation has become more available to patients with early HCC.

Screening has become accepted in clinical practice despite a lack of definitive data. In a survey, 84% of surveyed hepatologists in the United States routinely screened cirrhotic patients, using AFP in 99.7% and US in 93% [26]. An AFP and US done every 6 months for cirrhotic patients is an acceptable screening program; however, 25% in the previously mentioned survey preferred CT for screening. The screening practice usually does not differ for patients with cirrhosis from hepatitis C versus hepatitis B versus other causes of cirrhosis, including nonalcoholic fatty liver, alcohol, hemochromatosis, or α_1-antitrypsin deficiency. Cirrhotic patients with disorders carrying a lower risk of HCC (eg, Wilson's disease), however, might be screened less aggressively [26]. Screening for patients with chronic hepatitis C or B without advanced fibrosis or cirrhosis is not recommended.

Screening should be individualized. If a patient's cirrhosis is so advanced that no treatment would be offered, then screening is not indicated. Screening is indicated only if treatment or intensive follow-up of detected lesions is reasonable. Proposed guidelines for the management of detected lesions include the following [17]: lesions less than 1 cm are usually followed with repeat imaging in 3 months to determine lesion persistence or growth; lesions 1 to 2 cm are considered for biopsy or closely followed; and lesions more than 2 cm may or may not require a biopsy depending on the clinical setting, imaging characteristics, and AFP level. The protocol for elevated serum AFP levels in the absence of any suspicious lesion is unclear. Indeed, the precise cutoff level triggering any action is undefined. Some pursue imaging tests (MRI, CT) to detect lesions for mild elevation of AFP (>25 ng/mL) [22]. Others might repeat the AFP in 1 month for mild elevations (eg, 20–50 ng/mL), especially if other reasons for a burst of hepatic regeneration exist (eg, recent flare of chronic hepatitis B or C).

Prevention

Primary prevention of hepatitis C and B virus infection through control of high-risk behavior (eg, intravenous drug use), adequate screening of blood products, and vaccination are likely to be highly effective if such programs and policies were to be widely implemented. The annual incidence of hepatitis C infection has fallen in the United States since the 1970s, when intravenous drug use was more widespread and screening tests for hepatitis C were unavailable. The AIDS epidemic seems to have considerably decreased intravenous drug use. Posttransfusion hepatitis C has become exceedingly rare since the implementation of improved anti–hepatitis C virus antibody testing by American blood banks in 1992. A vaccine for hepatitis C remains elusive because of lack of host protective antibody and viral immune escape mechanisms.

The incidence of hepatitis B fell with the decline in intravenous drug use, and safer sexual practices caused by AIDS awareness. Available vaccine will significantly decrease the incidence of HCC related to chronic hepatitis B. Data from Taiwan suggest a decrease in HCC incidence in children with childhood vaccination against hepatitis B [27]. Presumably this will eventually produce a drop in the incidence of HCC in adults when the first cohort of vaccinated children reach adulthood.

Secondary prevention of HCC by control of viral replication and hepatic injury may be vital for the millions already chronically infected with hepatitis C or B virus. Treatment to eradicate or control the viruses decreases the chronic inflammation and regeneration of hepatocytes. In the United States, a large cohort has been infected with hepatitis C for 20 to 30 years; during this time period the risk of cirrhosis and HCC increases significantly. Treatment has improved significantly during the last several years. Combined therapy with a long-acting pegylated interferon-α injected once a week and ribavirin taken daily by mouth can achieve long-term eradication of hepatitis C virus in 40% to 70% of cases, depending on the viral genotype.

Eradication of hepatitis C virus infection should prevent progression to cirrhosis and decrease the risk of HCC. In a Japanese surveillance program of nearly 3000 cases of chronic hepatitis C followed since 1994, treated patients had a 50% reduction in HCC risk and patients with successful eradication of the virus had an 80% reduction [28]. In this uncontrolled study, treatment was significantly associated with HCC risk reduction in a multivariate analysis. Other studies support a decrease risk of HCC with treatment, and a meta-analysis by Camma et al [29] also points toward benefit. In another study, patients treated with interferon after HCC ablation had a decrease in HCC recurrence [30]. In the Hepatitis C Antiviral Long-Term Treatment against Cirrhosis multicenter trial, several hundred patients who did not respond to standard interferon and ribavirin therapy are being randomized to no treatment versus 42 months of interferon therapy for chronic suppression. One of the measured outcomes is HCC occurrence [31].

Treatment of patients for hepatitis C virus is hampered in cirrhotics by decreased tolerance to therapy, lower response rates, and unclear benefit in terms of lowering HCC risk [32,33]. Nonetheless, viral eradication may even benefit cirrhotics by slowing or preventing liver failure. Moreover, eradication before liver transplantation prevents recurrence of infection after transplantation [32]. Whether treatment or eradication in cirrhotics lessens the risk of HCC is undetermined, but studies clearly demonstrate that fibrosis and cirrhosis can regress after eradication [34].

Treatment for chronic hepatitis B continues to improve. Treatment options include interferon or the nucleoside analogues lamivudine and adefovir. Lasting seroconversion (ie, development of anti-HBe antibody and loss of HBeAg) may occur in 30% to 40% of patients treated with interferon for 4 to 6 months. Seroconversion is less likely and less stable with nucleoside analogue treatment, but these agents generally suppress viral replication. Even after viral mutation, which produces lamivudine resistance, viral replication can again be suppressed in 85% by adding adefovir [35]. Arguments for benefit and decreased risk of HCC are similar to those for hepatitis C virus treatment. Suppression of hepatitis B virus presumably results in less inflammation and hepatic regeneration, and decreased risk of integration of the viral genome into host DNA.

The available data suggest that hepatitis B virus treatment lowers the risk of HCC. Natural history studies suggest that decreased viral replication is associated with less risk of HCC. In one study of 11,893 Taiwanese men followed for 8 years, the relative risk of HCC was 60.2 for patients with both HBsAg and HBeAg in serum (indicating high viral replication) compared with 9.6 for those with only HBsAg [36]. A randomized controlled trial of interferon treatment in HBeAg-positive patients showed a significant decrease in HCC incidence in the treated arm during 1 to 12 years of follow-up (1.5% versus 12%, $P = .04$) [37]. A follow-up study of 165 HBeAg-positive patients treated with interferon reported a significantly lower relative risk of HCC in responders compared with nonresponders [38]. A meta-analysis, however, failed to show clear benefit [29]. Data on nucleoside analogues and their effect on HCC risk are lacking, and placebo-controlled trials will be difficult to perform because lamivudine has become part of standard care. One placebo-controlled study was stopped on interim analysis because lamivudine clearly slowed progression to cirrhosis [39]. Although numbers were small, the hazard ratio for HCC development was 0.49 (95% confidence interval: 0.22–0.90; $P = .05$) for lamivudine treatment. Because lamivudine or adefovir therapy is less likely to produce seroconversion than interferon, long-term nucleoside analogue treatment may be necessary to lower the risk of HCC.

Chemopreventive compounds and vitamins are being explored. Diets high in carotenoid compounds may lower the risk of HCC [40,41]. Other compounds that induce antioxidant enzymes (eg, dithiolethiones and isothiocyanates) or bind toxins (eg, chlorophyllin binding of aflatoxin) are under clinical investigation [42].

Treatment

Introduction

Treatment for HCC depends on the stage of the tumor and of the chronic liver disease or cirrhosis. The former dictates the chance of cure or response to therapy, whereas the latter dictates the tolerability of therapy. Intolerability to therapy is more common for HCC than for other cancers because HCC typically evolves in the setting of cirrhosis, which increases both operative and chemotherapeutic risks. Moreover, advanced liver failure creates significant baseline mortality unrelated to HCC. Despite these problems, aggressive therapy may be successful, particularly for patients with early stage HCC and well-preserved hepatic function. The appropriate therapy is controversial and can vary from center to center.

Surgical resection

Perioperative mortality for HCC resection used to be prohibitively high (15%–20%), but has decreased to less than 5% today because of improved patient selection and surgical techniques [43,44]. Surgical resection may be offered to patients with single-lesion HCC and well-preserved hepatic function (eg, Child's A cirrhosis). Patients with Child's B or C cirrhosis cannot tolerate loss of surrounding nontumerous hepatic parenchyma during a local resection. Even some patients with Child's A cirrhosis (eg, those with signs of portal hypertension or hyperbilirubinemia) cannot tolerate and are not candidates for local resection. Metastatic disease and gross vascular spread into the main portal vein or inferior vena cava (by the hepatic veins) are also exclusion criteria. Large tumor size is not an exclusion criterion, but large tumors mandate large resections leaving less functioning parenchyma behind. Liver volume estimates based on CT or MRI scanning are used to predict whether the hepatic parenchyma remaining after resection is adequate. In Japan, hepatic clearance of indocyanine green is used for this purpose. Retention of more than 14% of indocyanine green at 15 minutes indicates poor tolerability of significant resection [44]. Comorbidity, such as significant coronary artery disease and diabetes mellitus, may also militate against resection [45,46].

Improved imaging technology allows for better planning of the extent of resection. Some centers use intraoperative US to delineate the vascular supply to the tumor [44]. Intermittently clamping the portal vein and hepatic artery significantly decreases intraoperative blood loss [44]. Preoperative embolization of the portal venous branches supplying the cancerous segments induces hypertrophy of the remaining lobes [47]. These refinements in selection criteria and surgical technique argue strongly for referral for surgery to tertiary medical centers.

For patients meeting selection criteria, resection offers 5-year survival rates of 50% to 70%, rates comparable with that provided by liver transplantation, but about 60% to 100% have recurrent HCC at 5 years after resection [48,49]. Close follow-up for recurrence of HCC with imaging and AFP levels at least twice annually is necessary. Not all patients develop recurrent HCC, however, and those who do may still be suitable for liver transplantation, repeat local resection, or ablative therapy (see later). A Markov model suggested that resection followed by liver transplantation, when necessary, may be cost-effective [50]. Improvements in technique and patient selection have made resection a primary therapeutic option for HCC.

Liver transplantation

Before 1995, the transplant community had lost enthusiasm for treating HCC because of survival rates as low as 40% at 4 years. In 1996, Mazzaferro et al [51] published data showing that transplantation could have long-term survival rates similar to non-HCC patients if the tumors were few and small. Specifically, patients with a single HCC less than or equal to 5 cm or up to three HCCs each less than 3 cm on pretransplant imaging had a 4-year survival rate of 75%. These criteria are now used by UNOS in the United States [52]. These criteria constitute T2 stage in the tumor–node–metastasis (TNM) staging system, with T1 being one lesion less than or equal to 1.9 cm (Table 1). Patients with extrahepatic spread or vascular involvement detected on imaging (eg, portal vein invasion) are excluded from transplantation. Appropriate patient selection for transplantation is critical for a successful outcome.

Poor organ availability hinders application of transplantation. Before 2002, prioritization of transplant candidates was based on Child-Pugh score. Scores were gathered into four large UNOS status groups (status 1, 2A, 2B, and 3) and time on the waiting list determined the ranking within each group. Under this system, patients with less than or equal to T2 HCC were moved into a higher priority group (status 2B), but waiting time within the group remained a significant factor. For example, a patient with a newly diagnosed T2 HCC was listed as status 2B, but all 2B patients with more

Table 1
American Liver Tumor Study Group modified tumor–node–metastasis staging classification

Classification	Definition
TX, NX, MX	Not assessed
T0, N0, M0	Not found
T1	1 nodule ≤1.9 cm
T2	1 nodule 2–5 cm; 2 or 3 nodules, all <3 cm
T3	1 nodule >5 cm; 2 or 3 nodules, at least 1 >3 cm
T4a	4 or more nodules, any size
T4b	T2, T3, or T4a plus gross intrahepatic portal vein or hepatic vein involvement as indicated by CT, MRI, or US
N1	Regional (portal hepatis) nodes, involved
M1	Metastatic disease, including extrahepatic portal or hepatic vein involvement
Stage I	T1
Stage II	T2
Stage III	T3
Stage IVA1	T4a
Stage IVA2	T4b
Stage IVB	Any N1, any M1

Data from Bruix J, Sherman M, Llovet JM, et al. Clinical management of hepatocellular carcinoma. Conclusions of the Barcelona-2000 EASL Conference. J Hepatol 2001;35:421–30.

accrued waiting time were ranked higher. As waiting times lengthened through the late 1990s, intention-to-treat survival for HCC patients listed for transplant plummeted. In Italy, intention-to-treat 2-year survival decreased from 84% to 54% after 1996 when mean waiting time increased from 62 to 162 days [53]. Many patients had tumor progression beyond T2 while awaiting transplantation and were dropped from the waiting list. In the United States, the cumulative probability of list drop out by HCC patients was 25% per year in 2001 [54].

In 2002, the MELD prioritization system replaced the UNOS status groupings in part to minimize waiting time as a prioritization factor. The MELD score is based on three laboratory values (international normalized ratio, bilirubin, and creatinine). It had originally been designed to predict short-term mortality after transhepatic portal systemic shunt placement, but was subsequently shown to predict 3-month mortality for patients awaiting liver transplantation. The MELD equation generates an integral score from 6 to 40, with higher numbers indicating higher mortality and ranking. Waiting time is considered only if two patients had identical scores in their blood group. The MELD equation is complex, but on-line calculating is available through UNOS [55].

To accommodate the HCC patient, this system awarded 24 or 29 for patients with T1 or T2 lesions, respectively. Also, extra points are awarded for every 90 days listed to represent a 10% increase in risk of list drop out. The frequency of liver transplantation for HCC nearly tripled in the first year of the new priority system [56,57]. More than 85% of these HCC patients waited less than 90 days for transplantation. The average waiting time decreased from 2.28 years before the MELD system to 0.69 years under MELD.

The new system favored patients with HCC. Non-HCC patients with MELD scores of 24 to 29 had a significantly greater chance of dying or dropping off the list than HCC patients because they often had more advanced liver decompensation [57]. Also, the increase in transplantation for HCC magnified the effect of inaccurate imaging diagnosis on organ allocation [58]. For example, 14% of transplants performed for HCC had no evidence of HCC on explant histology in the first 8 months of MELD [59]. This misallocation occurred more often for small, single lesions (ie, T1). Moreover, retrospective data indicated that patients with T2 lesions were responsible for much of the poor intention-to-treat outcomes under the old system. Patients with T1 lesions had less than a 10% risk of drop out in the first year of waiting [60]. For these reasons, the assigned MELD scores were decreased to 20 and 24 for T1 and T2 lesions, respectively, in 2003. This revision decreased the proportion of transplantations performed for HCC from 21% to 14% [57]. The rate was only 8% before MELD.

Adult-to-adult, living donor related liver transplantation has increased in the United States and Europe in response to the organ shortage [61]. Donors are usually young, healthy individuals with a significant relationship with the recipient (eg, family member, friend). The right lobe or 60% of the donor liver is removed and both the donated portion and the 40% remaining in situ grows to more than 85% of the original volume within weeks to months. Living donor related liver transplantation fills a vacuum in liver transplantation. Patients with special circumstances that increase mortality and morbidity, which are not reflected in the MELD score, are well served by living donor related liver transplantation. Patients with HCC beyond T2 stage can fall into this category. They have a 40% to 50% 5-year survival after transplantation, which is an acceptable outcome in oncology. Arguably, living donor related liver transplantation should be offered to an appropriate recipient candidate if the donor is willing because a living donor related liver transplantation does not take organs from the deceased donor pool. Nevertheless, such cases must be weighed against the 1 in 300 mortality and the morbidity for young, healthy donors. Also, 5% to 10% of engrafted right lobes may initially fail (primary nonfunction). These cases are relisted for a deceased donor organ and do impact this limited resource. Currently, there is no consensus on living donor related liver transplantation use for more advanced HCC. Decisions are made on a center-by-center and case-by-case basis, but a multicenter National Institutes of Health–funded study is currently evaluating the indications, risks, and benefits of living donor related liver transplantation.

Emerging data suggest that hepatitis C virus patients have lower survival after transplantation than other patients [62]. This might affect transplantation for HCC because most cases in the United States are associated with hepatitis C. Hepatitis C infection uniformly recurs in the grafted organ.

Posttransplant hepatitis C has a highly variable course from rapid decline with liver failure within the first year to quiescent disease for more than 5 years. The course seems to have recently become worse, with approximately 20% to 30% progressing to cirrhosis within 5 years after transplant, possibly because of the increasing age of deceased donors [63,64]. Older grafted livers may poorly tolerate hepatitis C virus infection after transplantation. This trend could adversely affect the cost-effectiveness of transplantation for hepatitis C–related HCC. Some data further suggest that retransplantation for recurrent hepatitis C cirrhosis has poorer outcomes than for other indications for retransplantation [65].

The rules for organ allocation for patients with HCC continue to evolve [59]. The following represents the current status of diagnostic criteria and listing prioritization for patients with HCC [52]. UNOS diagnostic criteria for HCC are satisfied by histopathologic findings, but such tissue diagnosis is not mandatory. Short of biopsy, the lesion or lesions must be detected by US, CT, or MRI. In addition, at least one of the following must be present: a vascular blush of the tumor on CT or MRI, a serum AFP level of greater than 200 ng/mL, an hepatic arteriogram consistent with HCC, or prior local ablation of the lesion. UNOS also accepts the diagnosis of HCC without biopsy in a cirrhotic patient with an AFP level greater than or equal to 500 ng/mL, regardless of imaging findings. If these diagnostic criteria are met, then T2 cases may be upgraded to a score of 22. T1 cases no longer receive upgrades. Patients with HCC at stage T3 or more may be listed under their calculated MELD score without any upgrades. Centers rarely list such patients for deceased donor transplantation because of a higher risk of posttransplant recurrence and mortality, but may consider living donor related liver transplantation for these patients.

Percutaneous ethanol injection

Only 7% to 20% of HCC patients are candidates for curative surgical intervention because of advanced tumor stage or comorbidities precluding surgery. Local ablative therapies are important therapeutic alternatives in these other patients. Small HCCs (<2–3 cm) can be locally ablated by percutaneous, US-guided needle injection of ethyl alcohol. Alcohol causes dehydration and coagulative necrosis of neoplastic cells. Ablation can be performed on outpatients using local anesthesia. Needles are typically 22- or 21-gauge, with a single end-hole or multiple side-holes. At each session from 1 to 10 mL of 95% ethyl alcohol is injected. Some centers use general anesthesia when more than 10 mL is injected at one session. Alcohol creates a hyperechoic image allowing real time observation of the infused area.

The procedure is well-tolerated with very low complication rates. In a review of 1008 reported cases, no deaths occurred and only 2.4% had minor complications, most of which were treated conservatively [66]. The major side effect is pain [67]. A disadvantage is the multiple sessions required; a study from five different Italian centers reported approximately six sessions for 2-cm lesions, 10 sessions for 2- to 3.5-cm lesions, and 12 to 15 sessions for 3.5- to 5-cm lesions [68]. Sessions can be done once or twice weekly. Moreover, complete ablation of lesions larger than 2 to 3 cm is difficult. Although no evidence of tumor on follow-up imaging is reported for lesions less than 3 cm, the rate of local recurrence rises to 7% to 27% when lesions under 4 to 5 cm are included [68,69]. On histologic analysis residual tumor is seen in about 30% of lesions [70]. This therapy becomes inadvisable for lesions larger than 5 cm because of the number of required sessions and poor efficacy. Percutaneous ethanol injection (PEI) is generally recommended only for lesions less than 2 to 3 cm.

PEI has been compared favorably with local resection for small tumors. One Japanese cohort study reported similar 1-, 3-, and 5-year survivals for PEI versus hepatic resection for lesions less than 3 cm (100%, 82%, and 59% for PEI versus 97%, 84%, and 62% for hepatic resection; $P = .96$) [71]. Disease-free survival figures were better for the hepatic resection group, but did not reach statistical significance (63%, 30%, and 10% for PEI versus 76%, 45%, and 26% for hepatic resection; $P = .10$). Another cohort study from France demonstrated similar survival figures, but showed significantly better disease-free survival with hepatic resection over PEI [67]. Prospective, randomized, controlled data are needed to confirm these findings.

Radiofrequency ablation

Radiofrequency ablation (RFA) has evolved rapidly in the last several years because of promising clinical data and improved technology. HCC tumors are destroyed by thermal injury from electromagnetic energy delivered by RFA probes. The probes are significantly wider (14–17 gauge) than the skinny 22- to 21-gauge needles used in PEI. The probes are connected to an alternating current generator, which also has one or two large grounding pads applied to the patient's thighs. The probe is placed into the tumor under US guidance. The current is concentrated in a small area around the probe; tissue ions close to the probe move in alternating directions with the alternating current creating frictional heat.

Heating above 50° to 60°C for 4 to 6 minutes causes irreversible damage, but diffusion and maintenance of this heat throughout the tumor takes longer. A typical session lasts 10 to 30 minutes with target temperatures ranging from 55° to 100°C. Higher temperatures at the probe are necessary to diffuse sufficient heat throughout the tumor. The high temperatures can produce charring of tissue at the probe, which can hinder heat diffusion. Recent probes have cool tips with dual lumens that allow continuous infusion of saline preventing overheating of tissues nearest the probe. Recent probes also have several extendable prongs that are deployed circumferentially into the tumor, arranged in an umbrella or flower pattern (Fig. 2) [72]. Each prong applies current to significantly enlarge the area of necrosis. Removal of heat

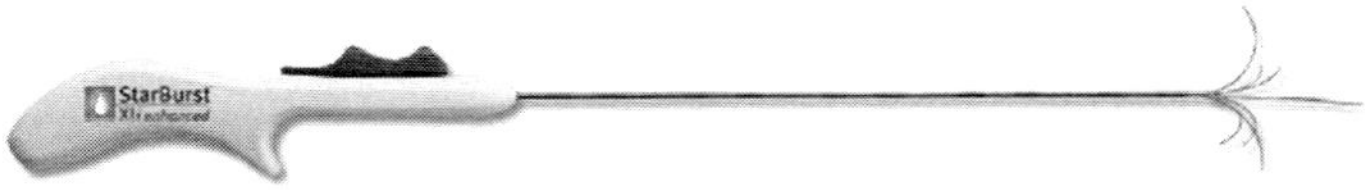

Fig. 2. Illustration of the StarBurst Xli-Enhanced RFA probe (Courtesy of RITA Medical Systems, Mountain View, California; with permission. Available at: http://www.ritamedical.com/products/starburstxli_enh.shtml#. Accessed April 15, 2004.)

by intratumor and surrounding vasculature can create a significant "heat sink," which limits thermal damage. Embolization of arteries supplying the tumor, by femoral artery access, has shown promise in extending tumor necrosis [73] but is not yet widely practiced.

Patient discomfort can be greater than for PEI because of the large probes and the longer intrahepatic therapy. Conscious sedation and occasionally general anesthesia are needed. The current and time settings are adjusted to obtain the desired area of necrosis, including up to 0.5 to 1 cm beyond the imaged border of the tumor. One capsular puncture of the liver is performed per session. Some centers admit patients overnight for observation postprocedure, whereas others release patients after several hours of observation. Complication rates are somewhat higher for RFA than PEI but are still acceptable. A large multicenter study reported a mortality rate of 0.37% (6 of 1610 patients) and major complication rate of 2.2% [74]. Only 0.5% had tumor seeding along the probe insertion track. Seeding may be prevented by heating the track during probe withdrawal. Certain tumors, such as those at the hepatic surface, have a higher risk of bleeding, peritonitis, or tumor spread. RFA is applied with trepidation in these cases, if at all.

Advantages of RFA over PEI include fewer sessions and higher rates of complete tumor necrosis. In a prospective study of tumors less than or equal to 3 cm, 1.2 sessions per tumor were needed to obtain complete ablation in 90% of tumors using RFA, compared with 4.8 sessions and an 80% complete ablation rate using PEI [75]. A randomized controlled trial from Japan comparing RFA with PEI for lesions less than or equal to 3 cm showed significantly fewer sessions required (2.1 versus 6.4) and fewer hospital days (10.8 versus 26.1) for RFA, with no significant differences in adverse events [76]. Two-year survival is excellent for both RFA and PEI (98% and 88%, respectively; $P = .138$), but local recurrence-free survival is better for RFA (96% versus 62%; $P = .002$) [77].

RFAs have higher complete ablation rates because of more uniform tumor cell killing including a 0.5- to 1-cm rim of normal hepatocytes surrounding the tumor. Ethyl alcohol tends to diffuse unequally through septated tumors. No margin of extended killing is obtained with PEI because ethyl alcohol tends not to diffuse into the surrounding cirrhotic liver. One study of biopsies of 33 tumors less than 3 cm, taken 4 days after RFA, revealed complete tumor necrosis and normal hepatocyte killing within the rimming margin for all specimens [78]. The only two cases of residual tumor occurred in completely excised specimens taken 4 weeks later. The foci of viable tumor cells were outside the RFA rim of ablation. Like PEI, RFA has difficulty ablating tumors greater than 3 cm, probably because of an inability to maintain high temperatures further from the probe. One study demonstrated complete necrosis by imaging in only 71% of 3- to 5-cm lesions and only 25% of lesions greater than 5 cm [79].

RFA has become the most popular ablative therapy because of higher efficacy in fewer sessions compared with PEI. Although no randomized controlled trials have compared RFA with surgical resection, RFA like PEI may yield comparable benefit with less morbidity and mortality.

Transarterial chemoembolization

Transarterial chemoembolization (TACE) has a niche in treating unresectable HCCs. It has higher efficacy with larger tumors (>3–5 cm). TACE takes advantage of HCCs 90% to 100% arterial blood supply, as opposed to the rest of the liver, which derives most of its blood from the portal venous system (only 20%–25% arterial) [80]. In TACE, the hepatic artery is accessed by the femoral artery under fluoroscopic guidance. Iodinated dye is administered to guide the catheter and provide a diagnostic angiogram.

Chemotherapeutic agents, including doxorubicin, cisplatin, epirubicin, and mitomycin, are mixed with lipoidal and delivered transarterially to the tumor. Some centers use a single agent, whereas others use a combination. The artery feeding the whole segment or subsegment harboring the tumor is usually selected. No single agent or combination has shown efficacy above others. Lipoidol is a poppy seed oil that preferentially stays in HCC tissue for days to weeks, increasing chemotherapy contact time. Immediately after delivery, the major feeding artery is embolized with substances, such as absorbable gelatin sponge or polyvinyl alcohol particles, to produce ischemic damage to the tumor, permit better penetration of the chemotherapy into cells, and to increase dwell time of the chemotherapy by reducing blood flow. Patients are admitted to the hospital after the procedure for overnight observation. Fever and a brisk rise in serum aminotransferase levels commonly occur the next day. If otherwise stable, patients are usually released with close follow-up and oral analgesics. The therapy can be repeated 8 to 12 weeks later depending on patient tolerance, angiographic findings, and follow-up imaging results.

TACE is generally only offered to patients with Child's A or B cirrhosis because the therapy injures surrounding hepatic parenchyma and results in decreased hepatic function. Patients with poor performance status, renal failure, poorly controlled ascites, or encephalopathy are often excluded. Usually, a platelet count greater than or equal to 50,000/mL and an international normalized ratio less than 2 is required. Patients with portal vein thrombosis are often excluded because of the risk of ischemia to large hepatic areas. In marginal candidates, superselective arterial cannulation of just the tumor-feeding artery and chemotherapy delivery without embolization can be performed to limit collateral damage. Even with these patient selection criteria and precautions, significant complications, such as hepatic decompensation and abscess, occur in 2.5% to 15% of cases [60,81,82].

Like RFA and PEI, TACE has better success with smaller tumors (<4–5 cm). One study demonstrated a 33% local recurrence rate at 4 years for tumors less than 4 cm [83]. Only 17% of tumors greater than 5 cm undergo complete necrosis [84]. The periphery of large tumors may have neovascularization with blood supply from other arteries (eg, phrenic, intercostals) or the portal venous system. These areas are less affected by TACE. Nevertheless, TACE can induce tumor necrosis (>80%) and slow growth in most large tumors [85]. Radiographic response rates can be as high as 80%. This represents the most practical nonsurgical option for patients with large HCC.

Until recently, studies showing improved survival after TACE were unavailable. In fact, a randomized controlled trial from France comparing TACE with symptomatic care failed to show survival benefit [86]. This study was criticized for an unusually high survival in the control group, an unusually high rate of liver failure in the treated group, and low study power [87]. Lo et al [88] in Hong Kong, however, showed improved 1-, 2-, and 3-year survival in the TACE group compared with untreated controls (57%, 31%, and 26% versus 32%, 11%, and 3%; $P = .002$). A Spanish study was truncated because of improved survival benefit for the TACE group on interim analysis (63% 2-year survival with TACE versus 27% 2-year survival with no treatment) [89]. TACE seems to improve survival based on these studies and a recent meta-analysis [90].

TACE offers improved survival to patients with unresectable HCC and mild to moderate hepatic decompensation. The procedure is performed by interventional radiologists in conjunction with oncologists who prescribe the chemotherapy. It is invasive, carries a higher risk than PEI or RFA, and requires hospitalization. It provides an important option for patients with tumors too large for RFA or PEI.

Systemic chemotherapy

Systemic chemotherapy for HCC has had disappointing results. HCC is believed to be relatively drug resistant. The multidrug resistant gene (*MDR1*) is active in HCC cells and hyperplastic hepatocytes [91]. HCC patients usually have underlying cirrhosis that decreases tolerability of cytotoxic agents. For example, cirrhotic patients often have anemia, leukopenia, or thrombocytopenia and are immunosuppressed and prone to infections. HCC patients referred to the oncologist usually have hepatic decompensation or advanced HCC. Others may have advanced age, poor functional status, or significant comorbidities that disqualified them from other therapies. It is not surprising that chemotherapy clinical trials have shown disappointing results.

Several chemotherapeutic agents, including cisplatin, etoposide, and epirubicin, have been tried for HCC. Doxorubicin (Adriamycin) is the closest to a standard chemotherapeutic agent for HCC. As a single agent, it has shown a modest survival advantage over no treatment [92], with a 25% overall response rate and median survival of 4 months [93].

Interferon-α has antiviral and antitumor activities, but is not effective as a single agent. It is often tried in combination with other agents. Of 50 patients with advanced unresectable HCC treated with a combination of cisplatin, doxorubicin, 5-fluorouracil, and interferon-α (abbreviated as PIAF) 13% had a partial response demonstrated by follow-up imaging [94]. Nine patients had sufficient tumor shrinkage to qualify for surgical resection. Of these nine, four had only necrotic tissue at the tumor site in the resected specimen. Toxicities included significant leukopenia in 34% and two deaths related to neutropenic sepsis. Growth factors were not administered, however, to increase the neutrophil counts. Overall median survival was 8.9 months, but 94% of patients were HBsAg positive with a median age of 47. Also, median Karnofsky score was 90%. There was no control arm. Randomized controlled data and data on HCV-related HCC are needed.

A phase III, multinational trial of thymitaq (nolatrexed dihydrochloride), which inhibits thymidylate synthase for unresectable HCC, is ongoing. Capecitabine is an orally administered prodrug of 5-fluorouracil. One preliminary study demonstrated a 13% response rate in HCC patients. Many patients (37%) developed hand-foot syndrome (palmar-plantar erythrodysesthesia), but therapy was otherwise well tolerated [95]. Other studied agents or hormones, such as tamoxifen, octreotide, and thalidomide, have less efficacy than doxorubicin.

Chemotherapy is theoretically appealing for the many patients who present with advanced-stage HCC or have contraindications for other therapy. Chemotherapy, however, remains disappointing. Indeed, supportive care without therapy may be reasonable for patients with advanced cirrhosis or poor functional status. Young patients with good functional status and early cirrhosis presenting with large, unresectable tumors should be considered for chemotherapy.

Treatment summary

Stage of tumor, degree of hepatic dysfunction, comorbidities, and functional status dictate which therapeutic options are reasonable. An overview of options is graphically depicted with TNM tumor stage on the ordinate axis and Child-Pugh stage on the abscissa (Fig. 3). Usually, curative options are restricted to those with early stage HCC (T1 or T2). Transplantation is the best option for T2 lesions. The Barcelona-Clinic Liver Cancer Group

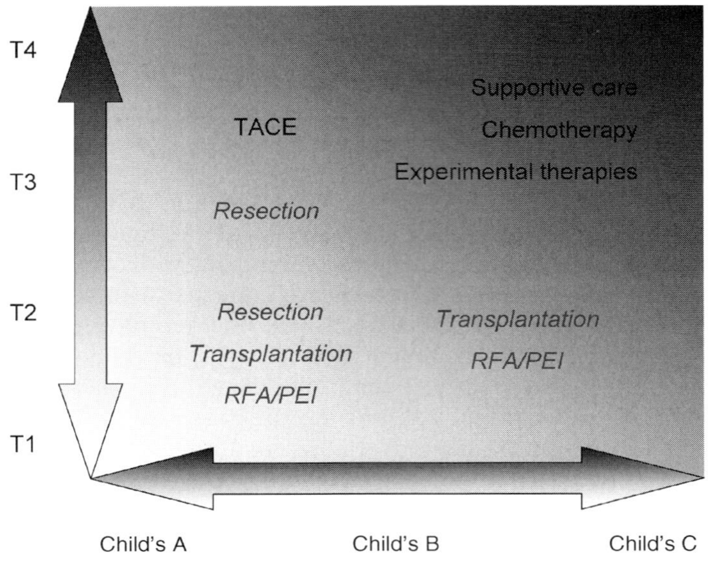

Fig. 3. Recommended HCC treatments plotted against the TNM (tumor, node, metastases) tumor stage and Child-Pugh status. Italicized treatments are potentially curative. PEI, percutaneous ethanol injection; RFA, radiofrequency ablation; TACE, transarterial chemoembolization.

provides a detailed therapeutic algorithm (Fig. 4) [96]. Patients are stratified by Okuda stage, Child-Pugh class, or performance status. Okuda stages 1 through 3 are based on tumor size, serum albumin level, presence of ascites, and serum bilirubin level, with 3 having more advanced disease [97]. Each major group is then subclassified by size and number of lesions and by extrahepatic spread of HCC.

Although treatment varies somewhat from center to center, the best option for early HCC and mild to moderate hepatic dysfunction (eg, no significant portal hypertension or hyperbilirubinemia) is controversial. Strong advocates for hepatic resection, RFA, and transplantation can be found. Liver transplantation eliminates the high recurrence rate by removing the entire liver and the MELD system has made it somewhat easier for HCC patients to be transplanted. Liver transplantation, however, brings measurable morbidity from life-long immunosuppression. Resection has an acceptable operative mortality and 3- to 5-year survival rates comparable to liver transplantation. Recurrences may be retreated, even with liver

Fig. 4. Algorithm for HCC treatment according to the cancer stage and the level of hepatic function. M1, metastatic disease; N1, regional (porta hepatis) node involvement; PEI, percutaneous ethanol injection; RFA, radiofrequency ablation; TACE, transarterial chemoembolization. (*Adapted from* Llovet JM, Bru C, Bruix J. Prognosis of hepatocellular carcinoma: the BCLC staging classification. Semin Liver Dis 1999:19;329–38; with permission.)

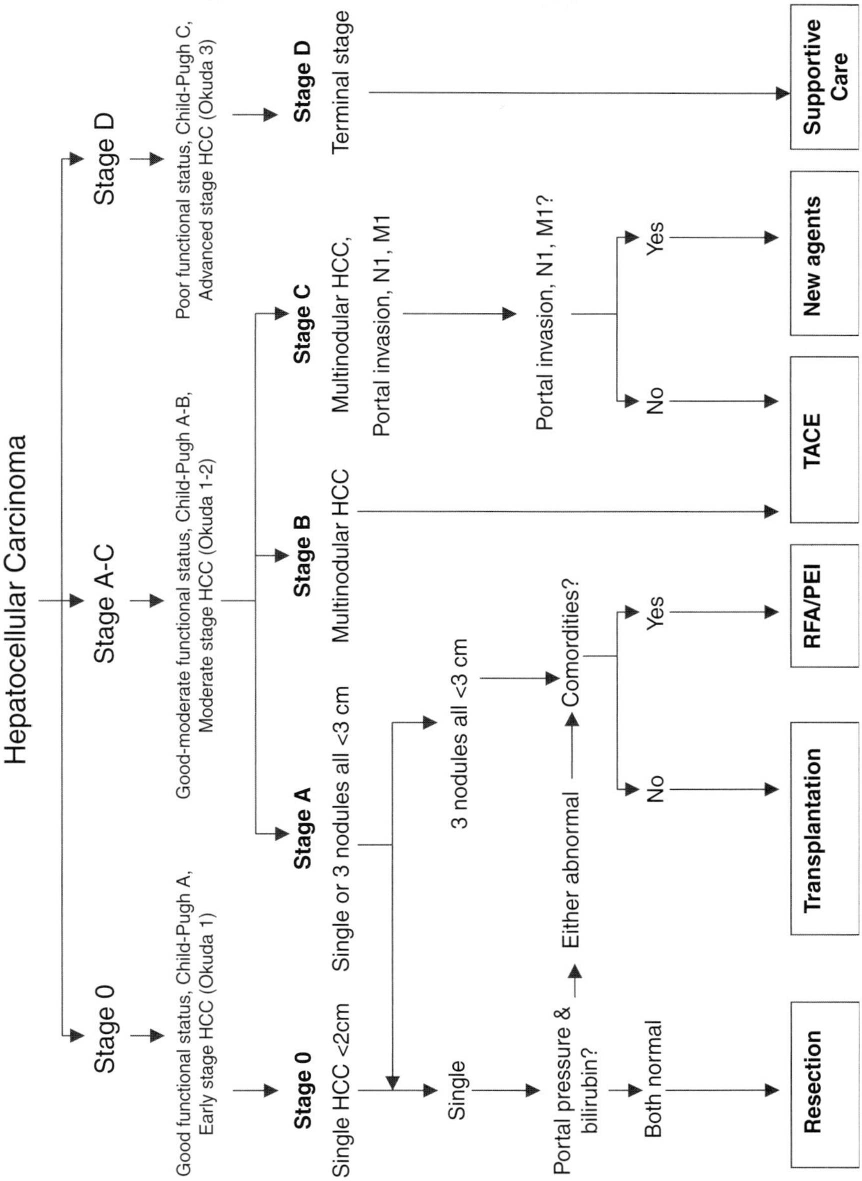
Hepatocellular Carcinoma
Stage 0
Stage A-C
Stage D
Good functional status, Child-Pugh A, Early stage HCC (Okuda 1)
Good-moderate functional status, Child-Pugh A-B, Moderate stage HCC (Okuda 1-2)
Poor functional status, Child-Pugh C, Advanced stage HCC (Okuda 3)
Stage 0
Single HCC <2cm
Stage A
Single or 3 nodules all <3 cm
Stage B
Multinodular HCC
Stage C
Multinodular HCC,
Portal invasion, N1, M1
Stage D
Terminal stage
Single
3 nodules all <3 cm
Portal pressure & bilirubin?
Either abnormal
Comordities?
Portal invasion, N1, M1?
Both normal
No
Yes
No
Yes
Resection
Transplantation
RFA/PEI
TACE
New agents
Supportive Care

transplantation. Conversely, if recurrence presents at greater than stage T2, then the opportunity for curative transplantation has been lost. RFA has a lower procedure morbidity and mortality than resection. The choice between the three options largely depends on the center. It is hoped that randomized clinical trials, particularly for RFA versus resection, will be forthcoming.

Summary

Much information has been gained in the diagnosis and treatment of HCC during the last 15 years. Ever improving imaging technology has made nonhistologic diagnostic criteria possible, albeit controversial. Liver transplantation, resection, and RFA are considered curative options. Yet, HCC incidence is steadily rising because of limited progress on disease prevention. Accurate and cost-effective screening is necessary. Presently, only 10% to 15% of HCC patients present with a curative stage of disease.

Because the field of HCC is rapidly changing, patients with HCC should be referred to liver centers with a full array of services, from surgical to oncologic. The prognosis for HCC patients will surely improve with a multidisciplinary approach to care and further clinical research. Better screening and prevention of recurrence should eventually improve survival. It is hoped that antiviral treatment studies will lower the risk of HCC, and that these changes will occur soon enough to help the many patients at risk for or diagnosed with HCC over the next several years.

References

[1] Szilagyi A, Alpert L. Clinical and histopathological variation in hepatocellular carcinoma. Am J Gastroenterol 1995;90:15–23.

[2] Di Bisceglie AM. Epidemiology and clinical presentation of hepatocellular carcinoma. J Vasc Interv Radiol 2002;13:S169–71.

[3] Kato Y, Tanaka N, Kobayashi K, Ikeda T, Hattori N, Nonomura A. Growth of hepatocellular carcinoma into the right atrium. Report of five cases. Ann Intern Med 1983;99:472–4.

[4] Gebo KA, Chander G, Jenckes MW, Ghanem KG, Herlong HF, Torbenson MS, et al. Screening tests for hepatocellular carcinoma in patients with chronic hepatitis C: a systematic review. Hepatology 2002;36:S84–92.

[5] Marrero JA, Su GL, Wei W, Emick D, Conjeevaram HS, Fontana RJ, et al. Des-gamma carboxyprothrombin can differentiate hepatocellular carcinoma from nonmalignant chronic liver disease in American patients. Hepatology 2003;37:1114–21.

[6] Capurro M, Wanless IR, Sherman M, Deboer G, Shi W, Miyoshi E, et al. Glypican-3: a novel serum and histochemical marker for hepatocellular carcinoma. Gastroenterology 2003;125: 89–97.

[7] Libbrecht L, Bielen D, Verslype C, Vanbeckevoort D, Pirenne J, Nevens F, et al. Focal lesions in cirrhotic explant livers: pathological evaluation and accuracy of pretransplantation imaging examinations. Liver Transpl 2002;8:749–61.

[8] Krinsky GA, Lee VS, Theise ND, Weinreb JC, Rofsky NM, Diflo T, et al. Hepatocellular carcinoma and dysplastic nodules in patients with cirrhosis: prospective diagnosis with MR imaging and explantation correlation. Radiology 2001;219:445–54.

[9] Hohmann J, Albrecht T, Hoffmann CW, Wolf KJ. Ultrasonographic detection of focal liver lesions: increased sensitivity and specificity with microbubble contrast agents. Eur J Radiol 2003;46:147–59.
[10] Fracanzani AL, Burdick L, Borzio M, Roncalli M, Bonelli N, Borzio F, et al. Contrast-enhanced Doppler ultrasonography in the diagnosis of hepatocellular carcinoma and premalignant lesions in patients with cirrhosis. Hepatology 2001;34:1109–12.
[11] Torzilli G, Minagawa M, Takayama T, Inoue K, Hui AM, Kubota K, et al. Accurate preoperative evaluation of liver mass lesions without fine-needle biopsy. Hepatology 1999;30: 889–93.
[12] Burrel M, Llovet JM, Ayuso C, Iglesias C, Sala M, Miquel R, et al. Barcelona Clinic Liver Cancer Group. MRI angiography is superior to helical CT for detection of HCC prior to liver transplantation: an explant correlation. Hepatology 2003;38:1034–42.
[13] Caturelli E, Ghittoni G, Roselli P, De Palo M, Anti M. Fine needle biopsy of focal liver lesions: the hepatologist's point of view. Liver Transpl 2004;10:S26–9.
[14] Livraghi T, Torzilli G, Lazzaroni S, Olivari N. Biopsia percutanea con ago sottile delle lesioni focali. In: Torzilli G, Olivari N, Livraghi T, Di Candio G, editors. Ecografia in Chirurgia. vol. 14. Milan: Poletto Editore; 1997. p. 167–90.
[15] Durand F, Regimbeau JM, Belghiti J, Sauvanet A, Vilgrain V, Terris B, et al. Assessment of the benefits and risks of percutaneous biopsy before surgical resection of hepatocellular carcinoma. J Hepatol 2001;35:254–8.
[16] Huang GT, Sheu JC, Yang PM, Lee HS, Wang TH, Chen DS. Ultrasound-guided cutting biopsy for the diagnosis of hepatocellular carcinoma: a study based on 420 patients. J Hepatol 1996;25:334–8.
[17] Bruix J, Sherman M, Llovet JM, Beaugrand M, Lencioni R, Burroughs AK, et al. Clinical management of hepatocellular carcinoma. Conclusions of the Barcelona-2000 EASL Conference. J Hepatol 2001;35:421–30.
[18] Yao FY, Ferrell L, Bass NM, Watson JJ, Bacchetti P, Venook A, et al. Liver transplantation for hepatocellular carcinoma: expansion of the tumor size limits does not adversely impact survival. Hepatology 2001;33:1394–403.
[19] Sherman M. Alphafetoprotein: an obituary. J Hepatol 2001;34:603–5.
[20] Everson GT. Increasing incidence and pretransplantation screening of hepatocellular carcinoma. Liver Transpl 2000;6:S2–10.
[21] Sarasin FP, Giostra E, Hadengue A. Cost-effectiveness of screening for detection of small hepatocellular carcinoma in western patients with Child-Pugh class A cirrhosis. Am J Med 1996;101:422–34.
[22] McMahon BJ, Bulkow L, Harpster A, Snowball M, Lanier A, Sacco F, et al. Screening for hepatocellular carcinoma in Alaska natives infected with chronic hepatitis B: a 16-year population-based study. Hepatology 2000;32:842–6.
[23] Yuen MF, Cheng CC, Lauder IJ, Lam SK, Ooi CG, Lai CL. Early detection of hepatocellular carcinoma increases the chance of treatment: Hong Kong experience. Hepatology 2000; 31:330–5.
[24] Tong MJ, Blatt LM, Kao VW. Surveillance for hepatocellular carcinoma in patients with chronic viral hepatitis in the United States of America. J Gastroenterol Hepatol 2001;16: 553–9.
[25] Sharma P, Balan V, Hernandez JL, Harper AM, Edwards EB, Rodriguez-Luna H, et al. Liver transplantation for hepatocellular carcinoma: the MELD impact. Liver Transpl 2004;10:36–41.
[26] Chalasani N, Said A, Ness R, Hoen H, Lumeng L. Screening for hepatocellular carcinoma in patients with cirrhosis in the United States: results of a national survey. Am J Gastroenterol 1999;94:2224–9.
[27] Chang MH, Chen CJ, Lai MS, Hsu HM, Wu TC, Kong MS, et al. Universal hepatitis B vaccination in Taiwan and the incidence of hepatocellular carcinoma in children. N Engl J Med 1997;336:1855–9.

[28] Yoshida H, Shiratori Y, Moriyama M, Arakawa Y, Ide T, Sata M, et al. Interferon therapy reduces the risk for hepatocellular carcinoma: national surveillance program of cirrhotic and noncirrhotic patients with chronic hepatitis C in Japan. IHIT Study Group. Inhibition of Hepatocarcinogenesis by Interferon Therapy. Ann Intern Med 1999;131:174–81.
[29] Camma C, Giunta M, Andreone P, Craxi A. Interferon and prevention of hepatocellular carcinoma in viral cirrhosis: an evidence-based approach. J Hepatol 2001;34:593–602.
[30] Shiratori Y, Shiina S, Teratani T, Imamura M, Obi S, Sato S, et al. Interferon therapy after tumor ablation improves prognosis in patients with hepatocellular carcinoma associated with hepatitis C virus. Ann Intern Med 2003;138:299–306.
[31] This Month from the NIH. HALT-C Trial. Hepatology 2002;36:792–3.
[32] Everson GT. Treatment of patients with hepatitis C virus on the waiting list. Liver Transpl 2003;9:S90–4.
[33] Crippin JS, McCashland T, Terrault N, Sheiner P, Charlton MR. A pilot study of the tolerability and efficacy of antiviral therapy in hepatitis C virus-infected patients awaiting liver transplantation. Liver Transpl 2002;8:350–5.
[34] Shiratori Y, Imazeki F, Moriyama M, Yano M, Arakawa Y, Yokosuka O, et al. Histologic improvement of fibrosis in patients with hepatitis C who have sustained response to interferon therapy. Ann Intern Med 2000;132:517–24.
[35] Perrillo R, Hann HW, Mutimer D, Willems B, Leung N, Lee WM, et al. Adefovir dipivoxil added to ongoing lamivudine in chronic hepatitis B with YMDD mutant hepatitis B virus. Gastroenterology 2004;126:81–90.
[36] Yang HI, Lu SN, Liaw YF, You SL, Sun CA, Wang LY, et al. Taiwan Community-Based Cancer Screening Project Group. Hepatitis B e antigen and the risk of hepatocellular carcinoma. N Engl J Med 2002;347:168–74.
[37] Lin SM, Sheen IS, Chien RN, Chu CM, Liaw YF. Long-term beneficial effect of interferon therapy in patients with chronic hepatitis B virus infection. Hepatology 1999;29:971–5.
[38] van Zonneveld M, Honkoop P, Hansen BE, Niesters HG, Murad SD, de Man RA, et al. Long-term follow-up of alpha-interferon treatment of patients with chronic hepatitis B. Hepatology 2004;39:804–10.
[39] Liaw YF, Sung JJY, Chow WC, Shue K, Keene O, Farrell G. Effects of lamivudine on disease progression and development of liver caner in advanced chronic hepatitis B: a prospective double-blind placebo-controlled clinical trial [abstract]. Hepatology 2003;38(Suppl 1): 262A.
[40] Yu MW, Hsieh HH, Pan WH, Yang CS, Chen CJ. Vegetable consumption, serum retinol level, and risk of hepatocellular carcinoma. Cancer Res 1995;55:1301–5.
[41] Clemente C, Elba S, Buongiorno G, Berloco P, Guerra V, Di Leo A. Serum retinol and risk of hepatocellular carcinoma in patients with Child-Pugh class A cirrhosis. Cancer Lett 2002; 178:123–9.
[42] Kensler TW. Chemopreventive strategies for hepatocellular carcinoma. Presented at the NIH Conference on Hepatocellular Carcinoma, Screening, Diagnosis and Management, National Institutes of Health. Bethesda (MD), April 1–3, 2004.
[43] Poon RT, Fan ST. Hepatectomy for hepatocellular carcinoma: patient selection and postoperative outcome. Liver Transpl 2004;10(2 Suppl 1):S39–45.
[44] Makuuchi M, Sano K. The surgical approach to HCC: our progress and results in Japan. Liver Transpl 2004;10(2 Suppl 1):S46–52.
[45] Miyagawa S, Makuuchi M, Kawasaki S, Kakazu T. Criteria for safe hepatic resection. Am J Surg 1995;169:589–94.
[46] Matsumata T, Taketomi A, Kawahara N, Higashi H, Shirabe K, Takenaka K. Morbidity and mortality after hepatic resection in the modern era. Hepatogastroenterology 1995;42: 456–60.
[47] Fong Y. Surgical resection for hepatocellular carcinoma. Presented at the NIH Conference on Hepatocellular Carcinoma, Screening, Diagnosis and Management, National Institutes of Health. Bethesda, Maryland, April 1–3, 2004.

[48] Shiina S, Tagawa K, Niwa Y, Unuma T, Komatsu Y, Yoshiura K, et al. Percutaneous ethanol injection therapy for hepatocellular carcinoma: results in 146 patients. AJR Am J Roentgenol 1993;160:1023–8.
[49] Belghiti J, Panis Y, Farges O, Benhamou JP, Fekete F. Intrahepatic recurrence after resection of hepatocellular carcinoma complicating cirrhosis. Ann Surg 1991;214:114–7.
[50] Majno PE, Sarasin FP, Mentha G, Hadengue A. Primary liver resection and salvage transplantation or primary liver transplantation in patients with single, small hepatocellular carcinoma and preserved liver function: an outcome-oriented decision analysis. Hepatology 2000;31:899–906.
[51] Mazzaferro V, Regalia E, Doci R, Andreola S, Pulvirenti A, Bozzetti F, et al. Liver transplantation for the treatment of small hepatocellular carcinomas in patients with cirrhosis. N Engl J Med 1996;334:693–9.
[52] United Network for Organ Sharing. Resources. Policies. Available at: http://www.unos.org/policiesandbylaws/policies.asp?resources=true. Accessed April 15, 2004.
[53] Llovet JM, Fuster J, Bruix J. Intention-to-treat analysis of surgical treatment for early hepatocellular carcinoma: resection versus transplantation. Hepatology 1999;30:1434–40.
[54] Yao FY, Bass NM, Nikolai B, Davern TJ, Kerlan R, Wu V, et al. Liver transplantation for hepatocellular carcinoma: analysis of survival according to the intention-to-treat principle and dropout from the waiting list. Liver Transpl 2002;8:873–83.
[55] United Network for Organ Sharing. Resources. MELD-PELD calculator. Available at: http://www.unos.org/resources/meldPeldCalculator.asp. Accessed April 15, 2004.
[56] Sharma P, Balan V, Hernandez JL, Harper AM, Edwards EB, Rodriguez-Luna H, et al. Liver transplantation for hepatocellular carcinoma: the MELD impact. Liver Transpl 2004;10:36–41.
[57] Wiesner RH. Liver transplantation for hepatocellular carcinoma: the impact of the MELD allocation policy. Presented at the NIH Conference on Hepatocellular Carcinoma, Screening, Diagnosis and Management, National Institutes of Health. Bethesda, Maryland, April 1–3, 2004.
[58] Hayashi PH, Trotter JF, Forman L, Kugelmas M, Steinberg T, Russ P, et al. Impact of pretransplant diagnosis of hepatocellular carcinoma on cadaveric liver allocation in the era of MELD. Liver Transpl 2004;10:42–8.
[59] Freeman RB. Liver allocation for HCC: a moving target. Liver Transpl 2004;10:49–51.
[60] Yao FY, Bass NM, Nikolai B, Merriman R, Davern TJ, Kerlan R, et al. A follow-up analysis of the pattern and predictors of dropout from the waiting list for liver transplantation in patients with hepatocellular carcinoma: implications for the current organ allocation policy. Liver Transpl 2003;9:684–92.
[61] Trotter JF, Wachs M, Everson GT, Kam I. Adult-to-adult transplantation of the right hepatic lobe from a living donor. N Engl J Med 2002;346:1074–82.
[62] Forman LM, Lewis JD, Berlin JA, Feldman HI, Lucey MR. The association between hepatitis C infection and survival after orthotopic liver transplantation. Gastroenterology 2002;122:889–96.
[63] Gane E. The natural history and outcome of liver transplantation in hepatitis C virus-infected recipients. Liver Transpl 2003;9:S28–34.
[64] Berenguer M. Host and donor risk factors before and after liver transplantation that impact HCV recurrence. Liver Transpl 2003;9:S44–7.
[65] Roayaie S, Schiano TD, Thung SN, Emre SH, Fishbein TM, Miller CM, et al. Results of retransplantation for recurrent hepatitis C. Hepatology 2003;38:1428–36.
[66] Livraghi T, Giorgio A, Marin G, Salmi A, de Sio I, Bolondi L, et al. Hepatocellular carcinoma and cirrhosis in 746 patients: long-term results of percutaneous ethanol injection. Radiology 1995;197:101–8.
[67] Gournay J, Tchuenbou J, Richou C, Masliah C, Lerat F, Dupas B, et al. Percutaneous ethanol injection vs. resection in patients with small single hepatocellular carcinoma: a retrospective case-control study with cost analysis. Aliment Pharmacol Ther 2002;16:1529–38.

[68] Livraghi T, Bolondi L, Lazzaroni S, Marin G, Morabito A, Rapaccini GL, et al. Percutaneous ethanol injection in the treatment of hepatocellular carcinoma in cirrhosis: a study on 207 patients. Cancer 1992;69:925–9.
[69] Shiina S, Tagawa K, Niwa Y, Unuma T, Komatsu Y, Yoshiura K, et al. Percutaneous ethanol injection therapy for hepatocellular carcinoma: results in 146 patients. AJR Am J Roentgenol 1993;160:1023–8.
[70] Shiina S, Tagawa K, Unuma T, Takanashi R, Yoshiura K, Komatsu Y, et al. Percutaneous ethanol injection therapy for hepatocellular carcinoma: a histopathologic study. Cancer 1991;68:1524–30.
[71] Yamamoto J, Okada S, Shimada K, Okusaka T, Yamasaki S, Ueno H, et al. Treatment strategy for small hepatocellular carcinoma: comparison of long-term results after percutaneous ethanol injection therapy and surgical resection. Hepatology 2001;34:707–13.
[72] Medical Systems RITA. StarBurst Xli-Enhanced RFA probe. Available at: http://www.ritamedical.com/products/starburstxli_enh.shtml#. Accessed April 15, 2004.
[73] Rossi S, Garbagnati F, Lencioni R, Allgaier HP, Marchiano A, Fornari F, et al. Percutaneous radio-frequency thermal ablation of nonresectable hepatocellular carcinoma after occlusion of tumor blood supply. Radiology 2000;217:119–26.
[74] Livraghi T, Solbiati L, Meloni MF, Gazelle GS, Halpern EF, Goldberg SN. Treatment of focal liver tumors with percutaneous radio-frequency ablation: complications encountered in a multicenter study. Radiology 2003;226:441–51.
[75] Livraghi T, Goldberg SN, Lazzaroni S, Meloni F, Solbiati L, Gazelle GS. Small hepatocellular carcinoma: treatment with radio-frequency ablation versus ethanol injection. Radiology 1999;210:655–61.
[76] Omata M. Chemical injection. Presented at the NIH Conference on Hepatocellular Carcinoma, Screening, Diagnosis and Management, National Institutes of Health. Bethesda (MD), April 1–3, 2004.
[77] Lencioni R, Cioni D, Crocetti L, Bartolozzi C. Percutaneous ablation of hepatocellular carcinoma: state-of-the-art. Liver Transpl 2004;10(2 Suppl 1):S91–7.
[78] Morimoto M, Sugimori K, Shirato K, Kokawa A, Tomita N, Saito T, et al. Treatment of hepatocellular carcinoma with radiofrequency ablation: radiologic-histologic correlation during follow-up periods. Hepatology 2002;35:1467–75.
[79] Livraghi T, Goldberg SN, Lazzaroni S, Meloni F, Ierace T, Solbiati L, et al. Hepatocellular carcinoma: radio-frequency ablation of medium and large lesions. Radiology 2000;214:761–8.
[80] Breedis C, Young G. The blood supply of neoplasms in the liver. Am J Pathol 1954;30: 969–77.
[81] Roayaie S, Frischer JS, Emre SH, Fishbein TM, Sheiner PA, Sung M, et al. Long-term results with multimodal adjuvant therapy and liver transplantation for the treatment of hepatocellular carcinomas larger than 5 centimeters. Ann Surg 2002;235:533–9.
[82] Spreafico C, Marchiano A, Regalia E, Frigerio LF, Garbagnati F, Andreola S, et al. Chemoembolization of hepatocellular carcinoma in patients who undergo liver transplantation. Radiology 1994;192:687–90.
[83] Matsui O, Kadoya M, Yoshikawa J, Gabata T, Takashima T, Demachi H. Subsegmental transcatheter arterial embolization for small hepatocellular carcinomas: local therapeutic effect and 5-year survival rate. Cancer Chemother Pharmacol 1994;33:S84–8.
[84] Fan J, Tang ZY, Yu YQ, Wu ZQ, Ma ZC, Zhou XD, et al. Improved survival with resection after transcatheter arterial chemoembolization (TACE) for unresectable hepatocellular carcinoma. Dig Surg 1998;15:674–8.
[85] Trevisani F, De Notariis S, Rossi C, Bernardi M. Randomized control trials on chemoembolization for hepatocellular carcinoma: is there room for new studies? J Clin Gastroenterol 2001;32:383–9.
[86] Groupe d'Etude et de Traitement du Carcinme Hepatocellulaire. A comparison of lipiodol chemoembolization and conservative management for unresectable hepatocellular carcinoma. N Engl J Med 1995;332:1256–61.

[87] Geschwind JF. Chemoembolization for hepatocellular carcinoma: where does the truth lie? J Vasc Interv Radiol 2002;13:991–4.
[88] Lo CM, Ngan H, Tso WK, Liu CL, Lam CM, Poon RT, et al. Randomized controlled trial of transarterial lipiodol chemoembolization for unresectable hepatocellular carcinoma. Hepatology 2002;35:1164–71.
[89] Llovet JM, Real MI, Montana X, Planas R, Coll S, Aponte J, et al. Barcelona Liver Cancer Group. Arterial embolisation or chemoembolisation versus symptomatic treatment in patients with unresectable hepatocellular carcinoma: a randomised controlled trial. Lancet 2002;359:1734–9.
[90] Llovet JM, Bruix J. Systematic review of randomized trials for unresectable hepatocellular carcinoma: chemoembolization improves survival. Hepatology 2003;37:429–42.
[91] Nagasue N, Dhar DK, Makino Y, Yoshimura H, Nakamura T. Overexpression of P-glycoprotein in adenomatous hyperplasia of human liver with cirrhosis. J Hepatol 1995;22: 197–201.
[92] Lai CL, Wu PC, Chan GC, Lok AS, Lin HJ. Doxorubicin versus no antitumor therapy in inoperable hepatocellular carcinoma: a prospective randomized trial. Cancer 1988;62: 479–83.
[93] Nerenstone SR, Ihde DC, Friedman MA. Clinical trials in primary hepatocellular carcinoma: current status and future directions. Cancer Treat Rev 1988;15:1–31.
[94] Leung TW, Patt YZ, Lau WY, Ho SK, Yu SC, Chan AT, et al. Complete pathological remission is possible with systemic combination chemotherapy for inoperable hepatocellular carcinoma. Clin Cancer Res 1999;5:1676–81.
[95] Aguayo A, Patt YZ. Nonsurgical treatment of hepatocellular carcinoma. Semin Oncol 2001; 28:503–13.
[96] Llovet JM, Fuster J, Bruix J, Barcelona-Clinic Liver Cancer Group. The Barcelona approach: diagnosis, staging, and treatment of hepatocellular carcinoma. Liver Transpl 2004;10(2 Suppl 1):S115–20.
[97] Okuda K, Ohtsuki T, Obata H, Tomimatsu M, Okazaki N, Hasegawa H, et al. Natural history of hepatocellular carcinoma and prognosis in relation to treatment: study of 850 patients. Cancer 1985;56:918–28.

ELSEVIER
SAUNDERS

Infect Dis Clin N Am
20 (2006) 27–45

INFECTIOUS
DISEASE CLINICS
OF NORTH AMERICA

Hepatitis B Vaccines

Andy S. Yu, MD[a], Ramsey C. Cheung, MD[b,c], Emmet B. Keeffe, MD[c,*]

[a]*Pacific Gastroenterology, 2101 Forest Avenue, Suite 106, San Jose, CA 95128, USA*
[b]*Department of Hepatology. VA Palo Alto Health Care System, 3801 Miranda Avenue, Palo Alto, CA 94304, USA*
[c]*Division of Gastroenterology and Hepatology, Stanford University School of Medicine, 750 Welch Road, Suite 210, Palo Alto, CA 94304, USA*

More than 350 million people worldwide are infected with the hepatitis B virus (HBV), and more than 1 million of them die each year of liver failure or hepatocellular carcinoma (HCC) [1]. The HBV prevalence varies widely from 0.1% to 20% in different geographic regions in the world, depending on the predominant age of infection and major mode of transmission [2]. There are currently 1.25 million HBV carriers in the United States, contributing to 17,000 hospitalizations and 5000 deaths annually [3]. As HBV is transmitted by body fluids, infection can be minimized by proper infection control practices, risk-reduction counseling, virus deactivation of plasma-derived products, and screening donors of blood, solid organs, and semen [4]. However the most effective way to prevent transmission of HBV is by immunization [5].

Indications

The national strategy to eliminate HBV transmission in the United States focuses on four major categories of subjects, including: (1) neonates, (2) infants, (3) adolescents, and (4) adults who are at increased risks for infection [6]. Identification of pregnant women who test positive for hepatitis B surface antigen (HBsAg) and timely postexposure prophylaxis of their newborns with hepatitis B vaccine can prevent most perinatal transmission

A version of this article originally appeared in the 8:2 issue of Clinics in Liver Disease.
* Corresponding authors. Liver Transplant Program, Stanford University Medical Center, 750 Welch Road, Suite 210, Palo Alto, CA 94304–1509.
E-mail address: ekeeffe@stanford.edu (E.B. Keeffe).

doi:10.1016/j.idc.2006.01.004

[7]. Hepatitis B vaccine is now recommended for all newborns before hospital discharge, regardless of maternal HBsAg status. Neonates born to mothers who are chronic HBsAg carriers should receive the first dose of vaccine within 12 hours of birth, accompanied by hepatitis B immune globulin (HBIG) at a different injection site. To further prevent transmission of HBV, both universal vaccination of infants and catch-up vaccination of all adolescents are now recommended in the United States (Box 1) [8]. It is required by 33 states for entry to middle school or seventh grade, three states for college entry, and by some colleges for matriculation. Juvenile correctional vaccination programs can also prevent infections among detainees [9].

Hepatitis B vaccine should be administered to adult populations at high risk for infection. High-risk ethnic groups include those who live in or emigrated from endemic areas, such as Asia and sub-Saharan Africa. Travelers to endemic regions for a prolonged period, defined arbitrarily as 6 months, should also be vaccinated. High-risk occupational groups include people who may be in contact with blood or body fluids. Workers in health care

Box 1. Indications for pre-exposure hepatitis B vaccination

Universal
- All infants
- All children and adolescents not previously vaccinated

On the basis of risk
- Illicit injection drug users
- Sexual partners of HBV carriers
- Men having sex with men
- More than one sexual partner in the previous 6 months; history of sexually transmitted disease (STD); or treatment in an STD clinic
- Household contacts, including cellmates
- People in occupational contact with blood or body fluids
- Hemodialysis patients
- Recipients of clotting factor concentrates
- Inmates of long-term correctional facilities
- Travel to endemic area > 6 months
- Clients and staff of institutions for the developmentally disabled

Adapted from Weinbaum C, Lyerla R, Margolis HS. Centers for Disease Control and Prevention. Prevention and control of infections with hepatitis viruses in correctional settings. Centers for Disease Control and Prevention. MMWR 2003;52(RR-1):1–36.

professions or institutions for inmates or mentally retarded people are typical examples. High-risk patients include those on hemodialysis or those who are chronic recipients of blood products, such as patients with hematologic disorders or bleeding diasthesis. Individuals with multiple sexual partners should also be vaccinated. Other high-risk categories include illicit injection drug users and household contacts of hepatitis B patients [9,10].

A number of studies suggest patients with chronic liver disease (eg, chronic hepatitis C) may have a worse natural history when co-infected with HBV [11]. Hepatitis B vaccines are safe and immunogenic in patients with mild-to-moderate chronic liver diseases, although immunogenicity is poor in patients with advanced cirrhosis [11]. Consensus panels convened by the National Institutes of Health on the management of hepatitis C issued the recommendation that patients with chronic hepatitis C receive vaccination with hepatitis B vaccine, as well as hepatitis A vaccine [12,13]. Although the Advisory Committee on Immunization Practices (ACIP) of the Centers for Disease Control and Prevention (CDC) recommends immunization of all people with chronic liver disease with hepatitis A vaccine [14], the committee has not issued a recommendation for hepatitis B vaccine for such individuals. The failure to recommend hepatitis B vaccination for these people may have resulted from less convincing data supporting a more severe outcome than is available in the case of superimposed hepatitis A in patients with chronic liver disease. However, as all patients with chronic liver disease may be at risk of a more severe course if infected with either virus, it seems reasonable to vaccinate these patients against both hepatitis A and B early in the natural history of their liver disease. Despite the lack of a formal recommendation from the CDC, this is common practice.

Besides newborn infants of HBsAg–positive mothers, other people exposed to HBV infection should receive postexposure prophylaxis (Table 1). Active immunization with intramuscular hepatitis B vaccine is the management of choice for previously unvaccinated subjects and has at least 70% efficacy in preventing HBV infection [15,16]. The first of the three vaccine doses should be administered within a relatively short period of time after exposure. Concomitant passive immunization with one dose of HBIG, preferably within 24 hours, may provide additional benefit despite no firm data substantiating this approach [17].

Postexposure prophylaxis varies according to the immune status of an exposed patient who was previously vaccinated. Postvaccination testing for antibody to HBsAg (anti–HBs) is usually performed for selected vaccinees 1 to 2 months after the completion of immunization. It is only necessary for those who are at increased risk of HBV infection as noted previously: health care workers, hemodialysis patients, household contacts of hepatitis B carriers, or infants born to HBV carrier mothers. It can also be considered for those vaccinees likely to have poor antibody response. Testing for anti-HBs is not recommended for follow-up after routine vaccination [18]. An exposed person who never received postvaccination testing after previous

Table 1
Postexposure prophylaxis for individuals exposed to hepatitis B virus

Vaccination and anti–HBs status of exposed person	Treatment when source is found to be positive
Unvaccinated	HBIG × 1, and initiate hepatitis B vaccine series
Previously vaccinated	
Known responder	No treatment
Known nonresponder	HBIG × 2, or HBIG × 2 and initiate vaccine series
Anti–HBs response unknown	Test exposed person for anti–HBs:
	If adequate, no treatment is necessary
	If inadequate, administer HBIG × 1 and vaccine
	Booster, recheck anti–HBs level in 1 month

Abbreviations: anti–HBs, antibody to hepatitis B surface antigen; HBIG, hepatitis B immune globulin.

Adapted from Weinbaum C, Lyerla R, Margolis HS. Centers for Disease Control and Prevention. Prevention and control of infections with hepatitis viruses in correctional settings. Recomm Rep MMWR 2003;52(RR-l):l–36.

immunization should be tested for the presence of anti–HBs. If anti–HBs is not detectable, immunoprophylaxis with HBIG and a second hepatitis B vaccine series intramuscularly can then be initiated. The strategy to test for anti–HBs only after exposure was found to be more cost effective than performing postvaccination testing on all high-risk vaccinees [19].

If an exposed individual is known to be a responder by postvaccination testing, defined as having anti–HBs $\geq$ 10 mIU/mL, additional immunoprophylaxis is not required. The immunologic memory of a vaccine responder for HBsAg appears to persist over a long period of time, independent of anti–HBs titer, after active immunization with hepatitis B vaccine [18]. On the other hand, if the exposed subject is known previously to be a nonresponder, immunoprophylaxis should be immediately initiated with one dose of HBIG and a second series of hepatitis B vaccine intramuscularly. For the exposed individual who was again a nonresponder after the second course of hepatitis B vaccine, a dose of HBIG should be given, followed by another dose in a month (Table 1) [8,20].

Prevaccination screening and isolated antibody to hepatitis B core antigen

Prevaccination screening may be cost effective when the expected prevalence of prior HBV infection exceeds 30% [10], such as in the high-risk adult populations for whom hepatitis B vaccine is indicated. Occasionally potential recipients of hepatitis B vaccine test positive for antibody to hepatitis B core antigen (anti–HBc) but negative for both HBsAg and anti–HBs. Isolated anti–HBc may be found due to suppression of HBV replication by hepatitis C virus in co-infected patients [21,22], or in the setting of low level infection with undetectable HBsAg but a positive HBV DNA by polymerase chain reaction (PCR). Alternatively, an individual with isolated positive anti–HBc may have cleared HBsAg and had detectable anti–HBc and anti–HBs, but subsequently lost anti–HBs. Finally, an isolated anti–HBc may be a false-positive result especially in a low-risk population [23,24].

Anyone found to have isolated an anti–HBc should be retested. A diagnostic algorithm can be used for those who are persistently positive for anti–HBc only [25,26]. To distinguish among the three possibilities mentioned previously (low-level HBV infection, prior immunity without detectable anti–HBs, or false-positive result), the patient may be given a single dose of hepatitis B vaccine with follow-up testing with a quantitative anti–HBs in 1 month. Should anti–HBs become positive in high titer indicating an anamnestic response [27], a convalescent state is proven and no further vaccine injections are necessary. On the other hand, if anti–HBs remains negative after the single dose of vaccine, HBV DNA should be tested by a PCR technique. If HBV DNA is detectable indicating a low level of viremia, the patient has HBV infection and further vaccination is not necessary. On the other hand, a negative HBV DNA in combination with undetectable anti–HBs would establish that the patient is not infected nor has been previously exposed, indicating the need to complete the three-shot vaccine series.

Immunogenicity

The HBsAg particle is the immunogen in both plasma-derived and recombinant hepatitis B vaccines. This envelope protein composed of several allelic subtype determinants but only one common group-specific determinant "a," which allows cross-protectivity among different subtypes [28,29]. Vaccinated subjects may have transiently detectable HBsAg in the serum within the first 24 hours. HBV vaccines stimulate active synthesis of anti–HBs conferring immunity. The first commercially available hepatitis B vaccine in the United States, licensed in 1981, was derived from chemically treated or heat-inactivated sub-viral particles that were obtained from plasma of chronic HBV carriers. Physician acceptance of these vaccines was initially impeded by the unfounded concern of the product carrying other blood-borne infectious agents [5]. Plasma-derived products still account for more than 80% of all hepatitis B vaccines used worldwide; however, in the United States the plasma-derived product has been completely replaced by recombinant vaccines.

Recombinant hepatitis B vaccine consists of nonglycosylated HBsAg particles that are produced by cloning the S gene via the yeast *Saccharomyces cerevisiae*. These newly synthesized HBsAg particles are then extracted from disrupted yeast cells, physicochemically purified, adsorbed on aluminum hydroxide, and preserved with thimerosal [10]. The first recombinant vaccine became available in the United States in 1986, and there are currently two approved products, Recombivax HB (Merck & Co., West Point,

Pennsylvania) and Engerix-B (Glaxo-SmithKline, Philadelphia, Pennsylvania) (Table 2). In addition, Recombivax HB is available as combination with hemophilus influenzae type b (Hib) vaccine (Comvax) for children. Furthermore, Engerix-B is available as combinations with hepatitis A vaccine (Twinrix) for adults, and with polio and diphtheria-tetanus-pertussis (DTP) vaccines (Pediatrix) for children. Concurrent administration of HBIG or other vaccines, such as Hib or DTP, does not interfere significantly with the antibody response to hepatitis B vaccine [10,30].

Only one among seven clinical series in the literature comparing the immunogenicity of Recombivax HB and Engerix-B is a prospective randomized double-blind trial [31]. In this multicenter trial of 460 healthy subjects between 39 and 70 years of age, either Recombivax HB 10 mcg or Engerix-B 20 mcg was administered as three standard intramuscular doses over a period of 6 months [32]. The geometric mean titer (GMT) of anti–HBs 2 months after the last vaccine dose was significantly higher in the Engerix-B group (840 mIU/mL versus 340 mIU/mL). The seroprotection rate, defined as anti–HBs titer $\geq$ 10 mIU/mL, was higher in the Engerix-B group but did not reach statistical significance (91% versus 85%). In a separate prospective randomized but single-blind study, the superior immunogenicity of Engerix-B was only demonstrated in subjects who were aged 40 or older (87% versus 81%) [33].

The immunogenicity of other HBV antigens, including HBcAg, remains ill defined. Addition of the pre-S components neither enhances the immunogencity of HBV vaccines nor circumvents any immunologic unresponsiveness to the S protein [34]. In a single-blind multicenter trial where volunteers were assigned to receive hepatitis B vaccines containing S protein and pre-S2 of various doses, the titers of anti–HBs that were achieved correlated with the dosage of S protein, and not of pre-S2. Furthermore, the titers of anti–HBs achieved in each vaccine group were higher in those

Table 2
Recommended dosages of licensed hepatitis B vaccines in the United States

	Recombivax HB		Engerix-B		Twinrix	
Age group (years)	mcg	mL	mcg	mL	mcg	mL
<19	5	0.5	10	0.5	—	—
11–15	10	1.0	—	—	—	—
>20	10	1.0	20	1.0	20	1.0
Dialysis patients and other immunocompromised hosts	40	1.0[a]	40	2.0[b]	—	—

[a] Special formulation.

[b] Two 1.0 mL doses administered at one site, in a 4-dose schedule at 0, 1, 2, and 6 months.

Adapted from Weinbaum C, Lyerla R, Margolis HS. Centers for Disease Control and Prevention. Prevention and control of infections with hepatitis viruses in correctional settings. Centers for Disease Control and Prevention. MMWR 2003;52(RR-l):l–36.

subjects who were younger (aged 20 to 39 years versus 40 to 59 years), supporting the importance of age in achieving durable immunity [35].

Routes of vaccine administration

Hepatitis B vaccine is traditionally administered intramuscularly, using a needle of 1.0 to 1.5 inches in length and 20- to 25-gauge in caliber. The preferred injection site is the deltoid muscle in adults and anterolateral thigh muscle in infants. Among 194 health care workers who received intramuscular buttock injections of hepatitis B vaccination, only 58% subsequently developed detectable anti–HBs titers [36]. This finding was verified by a prospective randomized trial where health care workers who received immunization in the arm achieved higher seroconversion rate of 93% and GMT of 1454 mIU/mL, as compared with those who were injected in the buttock. Among those who received buttock injection, the seroconversion rate (83% versus 72%) and the GMT (387 mIU/mL versus 85 mIU/mL) were higher with the use of 2-inch needles versus 1-inch needles [37]. Buttock injection makes intramuscular delivery of the vaccine difficult and should be avoided.

Intradermal injection of vaccine leads to very efficient antigen processing. It requires only 10% of the dose used conventionally for intramuscular injection and thus might offer a cost-effective advantage. However, data regarding the immunogenicity of intradermal vaccination, compared with the intramuscular route, remain controversial, and the long-term immunogencity of intradermal vaccine remains to be established [31]. Among 425 health care workers randomized to receive plasma-derived hepatitis B vaccines at doses of 2 mcg intradermally or 20 mcg intramuscularly, postvaccination GMT was significantly lower in the intradermal group [38]. In a group of hospital employees who were retested 2 years after a documented response to primary HBV vaccination, more subjects who had received intramuscular inoculations as compared with those who received it by the intradermal route maintained durable response (89% versus 64%), with GMT of 66.4 mIU/mL and 20.7 mIU/mL, respectively [39]. In a study using an accelerated scheme of hepatitis B vaccine over a 6-week period for post-exposure prophylaxis, anti–HBs seroconversion was achieved in significantly more patients who underwent the intramuscular than intradermal route (77% versus 45%). The investigators in this latter report discouraged the use of an accelerated low-dose intradermal schedule when rapid protection against HBV was desired [40].

In contrast, other clinical studies of intradermal hepatitis B vaccine reported some encouraging results in subjects who were nonimmunized as well as previous nonresponders to intramuscular immunization [41]. A trial of 50 health care workers who were randomized to receive either intramuscular or intradermal vaccine series yielded comparable seroconversion rates of 100% and 96%, respectively [42]. In another study of 1400 health care workers, protective anti–HBs titer was achieved in only 68% of subjects after the third intradermal dose of hepatitis B vaccine, but an additional dose of 2 mcg by the same route increased those with adequate protective titer to 89% [43]. Four doses of 2-mcg intradermal vaccines would still cost significantly less than three doses of 20-mcg intramuscular shots. Intradermal vaccine was also explored for use as a booster injection in individuals whose anti–HBs decreased to below 10 mIU/mL 3 years after the primary vaccination series. It was equally effective as an intramuscular booster injection in inducing an antibody response but was associated with more frequent local reactions, such as pain and discoloration at the injection site (42% versus 17%) [44].

Predictors of nonresponse

An anti–HBs level of $\geq$ 10 mIU/mL is regarded as a protective serum titer. Patients with certain clinical characteristics may have a lesser chance to sero-convert than others. In a retrospective multicenter cohort study of nearly 600 health care workers who underwent postvaccination testing for anti–HBs within 6 months after completion of vaccine series, five independent variables were identified by multivariate analysis as adverse prognostic factors for sero-conversion [45], These predictors included increasing age, male gender, obesity as reflected by body mass index, cigarette smoking, and use of Recombivax HB rather than Engerix-B. When subjects were stratified by vaccine brands, the adverse predictors included only age, body mass index, and smoking for the recipients of Recombivax HB. On the other hand, male gender remained the only negative predictor for the recipients of Engerix-B.

Other studies have confirmed the predictive roles of increasing age, male gender, smoking status, and obesity that may be alternatively represented by higher weight-height index [33,36,46–49]. Medical conditions that compromise the immune system may negatively affect the response to hepatitis B vaccine. In a cohort of homosexual males, low antibody response of anti–HBs $<$10 mIU/mL or nonresponse to hepatitis B vaccine occurred in seven of 16 patients infected with HIV compared with six of 68 HIV–negative vaccinees ($P = 0.002$). Furthermore, the median anti–HBs titers after immunization in the HIV–negative and HIV–positive responders were 205 and 15 sample ratio units, respectively [50]. Other risk factors for nonresponse include other conditions that may compromise the immune system, such as chronic cardiopulmonary disorders, renal failure, hemodialysis, and prior organ transplantation (Box 2) [51].

Nonresponse to hepatitis B vaccine may also be modulated by genetic factors. When a vaccine series of three doses were repeated in a study [48], all of the eight initial hyporesponders and eight of the 20 initial

Box 2. Risk factors associated with poor anti-HBs response to hepatitis B vaccine

Increasing age
Male gender
Obesity
Tobacco smoking
Immunocompromised from chronic disease

nonresponders mounted an appreciable anti–HBs titer. When nine of the 12 refractory nonresponders were sampled, six of them carried at least one of two extended major histocompatibility complex (MHC) HLA haplotypes B44-DR7-FC31 or B8-DR3-SC01. In contrast, only two of the 11 revaccinees sampled who responded to the second vaccine series carried these haplotypes, suggesting a genetic contribution to immuno-genicity [52]. In a large series of nearly 600 subjects who received a full course of hepatitis B vaccine, an analysis of HLA haplotypes among the 20 vaccinees with the lowest anti–HBs titer responses indicated a disproportionately higher number of HLA-B8-DR3-SC01 [53]. When nine of the haplotype carriers were given three additional doses of vaccine, four of the five homozygotes but none of the nine heterozygotes remained hyporesponders. These findings implicate a recessive MHC–linked trait as a cause of hyporesponse to hepatitis B vaccination [53].

Efficacy of hepatitis B vaccines

Seroprotective rate up to 95% or above has been demonstrated in multiple placebo-controlled, randomized double-blind trials involving health care workers [29] and homosexual males [54–56]. This is defined as percentage of vacinees achieving an anti-HBs titer > 10 mIU/mL. Infection rates in reported studies were <4% among the vaccinees, in contrast with rates of 10% to 27% in the placebo arms. A significant reduction of hepatitis B cases within 75 days after randomization of subjects suggested the effectiveness of vaccine even when given shortly after exposure to the virus [55].

Patients who develop seroprotective titers will continue to maintain high levels of protection from clinical disease for at least a decade. In a large cohort of Yupik Eskimos who had a 94% rate of anti–HBs seroconversion, 76% maintained titers ≥ 10 mIU/mL after 10 years of follow-up. None became chronically infected despite development of anti–HBc in 10 vaccine responders, implicating subclinical exposure to HBV among vaccinees with durable protection against the virus [57,58]. Long-term follow-up in similar series have noted boosts in anti–HBs titers despite no interim booster vaccine injection, probably attributable to immunologic protection against viral exposure [59]. The maximal anti–HBs response postvaccination is strongly predictive of titer persistence and inversely correlated with the risk of viral infection, as demonstrated by a longitudinal follow-up of nearly 800 homosexual males for 5 years after vaccination [60].

A two-dose vaccine regimen over a 6-month period may suffice in producing a comparable long-term protection against HBV in immunocompetent hosts. In a group of young healthy adults who received Recombivax HB doses of 10 mcg or 20 mcg, anti–HBs seroconversion rates of 46% to 67% were observed after the first dose, but increased to 97% to 99% after the second dose with booster responses in GMT. Furthermore, a sizable proportion (75% to 89%) of vaccinees maintained titers $\geq$ 10 mIU/mL 2 years after the regimen was given, with 79% to 87% demonstrating rapid and vigorous anamnestic response after another booster dose [61]. Nevertheless, if immediate short-term immunologic protection is also desired, a three-dose regimen remains the preferred choice for individuals who are at high risk for infection during the initial 6-month period.

A few investigators have reported that the interval between the second and third vaccine doses is important in determining the ultimate anti–HBs titer. The CDC observed a significant rise in anti–HBs titers in those who received the third vaccine dose late (>7 months after the first dose) among the 1000 Yucpa Indian vaccinees [46]. Similar conclusion was drawn by an interesting study comparing the efficacies of three vaccine regimens, given at 0, 1, 2, 12 months; 0, 1, 6 months; and 0, 1, 12 months [62]. Booster anti–HBs responses were seen after the third dose for each of the last two regimens but were not observed until after the fourth dose in the first regimen. Furthermore, the ultimate titers achieved by the first and third regimens were comparable but 20 fold higher than that achieved by the second regimen with the third and last dose administered at 6 months. Hence, the anti–HBs response after a typical three-dose hepatitis B vaccine series depends on the time interval between the last two doses [62].

Anti–HBs seroconversion is appreciably lower with vaccination of immuno-compromised patients, such as those on hemodialysis, despite early reports of excellent results [63]. Suboptimal results with intramuscular double-dosing regimen prompt continued search for better solution. In a randomized double-blind placebo-controlled trial of double-dosed hepatitis B vaccine, only 63% of hemodialysis patients developed adequate antibody response [64]. This figure, however, decreased to 50% after correction for possible transfer of antibodies by blood transfusion. When compared with the placebo arm, there was no significant reduction in HBV infection within the first two years among the vaccinees (6.4% versus 5.4%) [64]. Similarly, the seroconversion rate with immunizing cirrhotic patients awaiting liver transplantation was dismal. Vaccinating these patients with standard doses produced seroconversion rate of 28%, compared with 97% achieved by healthy controls [65]. Even when a double dose was given to cirrhotic patients, the seroconversion rate was 44% and increased to only 62% with a repeat series [66].

Perinatal immunoprophylaxis with hepatitis B vaccine is now routinely given to newborn infants, with an additional early dose of HBIG for those who are born to HBV–infected mothers. The use of HBIG alone does not provide long-term protection against the infection [16]. The vaccine series should be initiated within the first 12 hours after birth for neonates born to HBsAg–positive mothers but may be administered by a relatively flexible schedule to those born to HBsAg–negative women [67]. With immunization, more than 95% of babies develop anti–HBs titer $\geq$ 10 mIU/mL [68,69]. Vaccinated infants of HBsAg–positive mothers should then be tested for HBV status at 12 months of age. Without immunization, >90% would be chronically infected due to vertical transmission of HBV [7]. As for adult vaccinees, hepatitis B vaccine affords long-term protection for most infants when initiated soon after birth [16,70], Even if children lose detectable anti–HBs later on in life, which occurs in up to half of individuals, a booster vaccine injection will almost always lead to a robust anam-nestic response and resurgence of anti–HBs [71–73].

A delay in the initial dose of vaccine increases the risk to the child for HBV infection [74], In addition, infants may fail immunoprophylaxis due to in utero infection, genetically determined nonresponsiveness, or vaccine-breakthough mutations in mother or in infants [5]. In utero infection of the fetus is relatively uncommon [75] but may result from placental leakage [76,77]. Vaccine-breakthrough mutations are attributable to immune pressure from either hepatitis B vaccine or HBIG [78] and may involve point substitution from glycine to argi-nine at codon 145 (G145R), asparagine to threonine at codon 126 (N126T), or asparagine to isoleucine substitution at codon 126 (N1261) in the S gene [79], plus many others that were discovered subsequently [80]. In general, the S gene mutation causes decreased binding of anti–HBs to determinant "a," thus allowing the mutant virus to escape neutralization [2].

The global impact of hepatitis B vaccination, including a decreased prevalence of chronic infection and associated complications, is clearly demonstrated in recent studies. In July 1984, Taiwan became the first country to launch a universal newborn hepatitis B vaccination program. Over the subsequent 15 years, a serologic survey of the prevalence of HBsAg among youngsters of ages 15 years or less demonstrated a significant reduction from 9.8% to 0.7%. In addition, seropositivity for anti–HBc, which reflects HBV infection and not vaccination, dropped from 20.6% to 2.9% [81]. A retrospective review in 1997 showed a significant decline in the average annual incidence of HCC per 100,000 children of ages 6 to 14 years, with 0.70 between 1981 and 1986, 0.57 between 1986 and 1990, and 0.36 between 1990 and 1994 [82]. Furthermore, the incidence of HCC in children of ages 6 to 9 declined per 100,000 from 0.52 for those who were born between 1974 and 1984 to 0.13 for those who were born between 1984 and 1986 [82]. On the other hand, the prevalence of S gene mutations among HBsAg–positive children has been increasing, from 7.8% in 1984 immediately before implementation of the universal vaccination program, to 19.6% in 1989 and 28.1% in 1994 [83]. It was not until 1991 in the United States that the ACIP recommended universal hepatitis B vaccination of all infants [6]. Shortly afterward the American Academy of Pediatrics and the American Academy of Family Physicians published similar recommendations. Nevertheless, in 1999 the proportion of children <3 years of age who were immunized against HBV had not yet reached the target of 90% as originally proposed by the Childhood Immunization Initiative [84].

Vaccine nonresponse and its management

Among individuals who do not respond to the initial series of hepatitis B vaccine, half may convert after an additional one to three doses [60,85]. Hypo-responders are more likely to seroconvert than nonresponders [86]. The use of investigational mix-particle vaccines containing pre-Sl, pre-S2, and S subunits does not enhance the seroconversion rate achieved by a standard S-unit vaccine of equivalent dosage [87]. Likewise, doubling administered doses for revaccination does not confer any immunologic advantage [88]. Nonresponders to a second series of vaccination are unlikely to develop adequate anti–HBs titers with further vaccine doses [5]. Another potential alternative is the use of vaccine adjuvants to enhance the immunogenicity of existing vaccines [89,90]. Clinical algorithms to reimmunize nonresponders have been described [86].

The use of granulocyte-macrophage colony stimulating factor (GM-CSF) as vaccine adjuvant operates by enhancing memory cell generation via both T and B cell activation; activating macrophages and other effector cells; increasing major histocompatibility complex (MHC) class II antigen expression on the surface of macrophages; promoting dendritic cell maturation and migration, upregulating co-stimulatory molecules on dendritic cells; accelerating the maturation of hematopoietic progenitor cells in bone marrow; and inducing localized inflammation at the site of injection [91,92]. Sixty healthy nonresponders to hepatitis B vaccine were randomized to receive intramuscularly high-dose Recombivax HB 40 mcg × three doses alone versus three injections of GM-CSF with each followed immediately in the same site by standard Recombivax HB at 10 mcg. Each arm produced an equivalent seroprotection rate of approximately 50% [93].

The nonresponse of renal failure patients to hepatitis B vaccine is due to immunosuppression attributable to uremia, inadequate dialysis, use of low biocompatibility dialysis material, hyperparathyroidism, anemia, iron overload, and malnutrition [94]. Efficient hemodialysis may significantly improve the response to vaccination [95]. In a pilot study of vaccine-naïve hemodialysis patients randomized to receive GM-CSF followed 24 hours later by one standard vaccine dose versus three monthly double doses of vaccine alone, superior seroprotection rate was achieved in the GM-CSF group (87.5% versus 25%) [96]. Impressive results of GM-CSF were noted in a separate trial in which it was used as a high-dose 150-mcg adjuvant before a four-dose hepatitis B vaccine series, resulting in a seroprotective rate of 100% at 7 months [97]. When used in hemodialysis patients who were nonresponders to previous vaccine series, GM-CSF as an adjuvant had variable results, significantly increasing the seroconversion rate and anti–HBs titers in some trials [98,99], but not in others [100]. Dose-dependent adverse events were documented with GM-CSF, including fatigue, nausea, rigors, and hypotension [101]. It is possible that other adjuvants, such as MF59 that has been used in influenza vaccines, may also increase the immunogenicity of hepatitis B vaccines.

Adverse effects of hepatitis B vaccines

Both plasma and recombinant vaccines are equally well tolerated [5,10,102]. Transient tenderness or pain may occur in up to a fifth of the vaccinees. Low-grade fever is found in $< 5\%$ of the cases. Other much less common adverse events, including fatigue, headache, malaise, nausea, dizziness, skin rash, arthralgia, myalgia, and respiratory distress, occur in $< 1\%$ of cases [5,103]. Anaphy-laxis may rarely occur, and epinephrine should be available for immediate use [10]. Among 850,000 vaccinees monitored by the CDC and Food and Drug Administration, 41 neurologic adverse events were reported, including Bell's palsy in 10, Guillain-Barré syndrome in nine, convulsions in five, lumbar radiculopathy in five, optic neuritis in five, transverse myelitis in four, and brachial plexus neuropathy in three. However, no conclusive epidemiologic association could be established between any neurologic events and the vaccine [104,105]. As animal reproduction studies have not been conducted with the vaccine, whether it can cause fetal harm when administered to a pregnant woman is unknown.

Immunotherapy using hepatitis B vaccine

Hepatitis B vaccine may serve as an immunomodulator for suppressing viral replication. In a study of the therapeutic efficacy of hepatitis B vaccine, 118 treatment-naïve patients with histologically and virologically proven chronic hepatitis B were randomized to receive either placebo or intramuscular hepatitis B vaccine in the form of S vaccine alone or combined pre-S2 and S vaccine [106]. After five vaccine injections were given, there was a significant but transient 6-month decrease in viral load that did not occur in controls, despite persistence of HBsAg in all patients. For the first time, hepatitis B vaccine was shown to decrease viral replication, which may pave the road for new therapies based on the concept of specific immunomodulation.

Summary

Immunization is the most effective way to prevent transmission of HBV and, hence, the development of acute or chronic hepatitis B. The national strategy to eliminate transmission of the virus in the United States includes vaccination of all newborn infants, children, adolescents, and high-risk adults. Postexposure prophylaxis is also advocated, depending on the vaccination and anti–HBs status of the exposed person. Seroprotection after vaccination, defined as anti–HBs $\geq$ 10 mIU/mL, is achieved in over 95% of all vaccinees. The hepatitis B vaccines are very well tolerated with usually minimal adverse effects. Predictors of non-response include increasing age, male gender, obesity, tobacco smoking, and immunocompromising chronic disease. For those who remain nonresponders after the second series of vaccination, adjuvants such as GM-CSF may be considered, but their results are variable.

References

[1] Lee WM. Hepatitis B virus infection. N Engl J Med 1997;337(24):1733–45.

[2] Lok ASF, Conjeevaram HS. Hepatitis B. In: Schiff ER, Sorrell MF, Maddrey WC, editors. Schiff's diseases of the liver. 9th edition. Philadelphia: Lippincott Williams & Wilkins; 2003. p. 763–806.

[3] Mover LA, Mast EE. Hepatitis B: virology, epidemiology, disease, and prevention, and an overview of viral hepatitis. Am J Prev Med 1994;10(Suppl):45–55.

[4] Alter MJ. Epidemiology and prevention of hepatitis B. Semin Liver Dis 2003;23(1):39–46.

[5] Koff RS. Vaccines and hepatitis B. Clin Liver Dis 1999;3(2):417–28.

[6] Centers for Disease Control and Prevention. Hepatitis B virus: a comprehensive strategy for eliminating transmission in the United States through universal childhood vaccination. Recommendations of the Immunization Practices Advisory Committee (ACIP). MMWR 1991;40(RR-13):1–25.

[7] Stevens CE, Taylor PE, long MJ, Toy PT, Vyas GN, Nair ON, et al. Yeast-recombinant hepatitis B vaccine: efficacy with hepatitis B immune globulin in prevention of perinatal hepatitis B virus transmission. JAMA 1987;257:2612–6.

[8] Centers for Disease Control. Inactivated hepatitis B virus vaccine. MMWR 1982;31(24): 317–28.

[9] Weinbaum C, Lyerla R, Margolis HS. Centers for Disease Control and Prevention. Prevention and control of infections with hepatitis viruses in correctional settings. MMWR Recomm Rep 2003;52(RR-1):1–36.

[10] Lemon SM, Thomas DL. Vaccines to prevent viral hepatitis. N Engl J Med 1997;336(3): 196–204.

[11] Keeffe EB. Acute hepatitis A and B in patients with chronic liver disease: prevention through vaccination. Am J Med 2005;118:21S–7S.

[12] National Institutes of Health Consensus Development Conference Panel statement. Management of hepatitis C. Hepatology 1997;26(Suppl 1):2S–10S.

[13] National Institutes of Health Consensus Development Conference statement. Management of hepatitis C: 2002 – June 10–12, 2002. Hepatology 2002;36(Suppl 1):S3–20.

[14] Centers for Disease Control and Prevention. Prevention of hepatitis A through active or passive immunization: recommendations of the Advisory Committee on Immunization Practices (ACIP). MMWR 1999;48:1–37.

[15] Xu ZY, Liu CB, Francis DP, Purcell RH, Gun ZL, Duan SC, et al. Prevention of perinatal acquisition of hepatitis B virus carriage using vaccine: preliminary report of a randomized, double-blind placebo-controlled and comparative trial. Pediatrics 1985;76(5):713–8.
[16] Xu ZY, Duan SC, Margolis HS, Purcell RH, Ou-Yang PY, Coleman PJ, et al. Long-term efficacy of active postexposure immunization of infants for prevention of hepatitis B virus infection. United States–People's Republic of China Study Group on Hepatitis B. J Infect Dis 1995;171(1):54–60.
[17] Beasley RP, Hwang LY, Stevens CE, Lin CC, Hsieh FJ, Wang KY, et al. Efficacy of hepatitis B immune globulin for prevention of perinatal transmission of the hepatitis B virus carrier state: final report of a randomized double-blind, placebo-controlled trial. Hepatology 1983;3(2):135–41.
[18] West DJ, Calandra GB. Vaccine induced immunologic memory for hepatitis B surface antigen: implications for policy on booster vaccination. Vaccine 1996;14(11):1019–27.
[19] Alimonos K, Nafziger AN, Murray J, Bertino JS Jr. Prediction of response to hepatitis B vaccine in health care workers: whose titers of antibody to hepatitis B surface antigen should be determined after a three-dose series, and what are the implications in terms of cost-effectiveness? Clin Infect Dis 1998;26(3):566–71.
[20] Centers for Disease Control and Prevention. Updated US Public Health Service guidelines for the management of occupational exposures to HBV, HCV, and HIV and recommendations for post-exposure prophylaxis. MMWR Recomm Rep 2001;50(44–11):1–42.
[21] Berger A, Doerr HW, Rabenau HF, Weber B. High frequency of HCV infection in individuals with isolated antibody to hepatitis B core antigen. Intervirology 2000;43(2):71–6.
[22] Weber B, Melchior W, Gehrke R, Doerr HW, Berger A, Rabenau H. Hepatitis B virus markers in anti-HBc only positive individuals. J Med Virol 2001;64(3):312–9.
[23] Schifman RB, Rivers SL, Sampliner RE, Krammes JE. Significance of isolated hepatitis B core antibody in blood donors. Arch Intern-Med 1993;153(19):2261–6.
[24] Silva AE, McMahon BJ, Parkinson AJ, Sjogren MH, Hoofnagle JH, Di Bisceglie AM. Hepatitis B virus DNA in persons with isolated antibody to hepatitis B core antigen who subsequently received hepatitis B vaccine. Clin Infect Dis 1998;26(4):895–7.
[25] Lau DT, Hewlett AT. Screening for hepatitis A and B antibodies in patients with chronic liver disease. Am J Med 2005;118:28S–33S.
[26] McMahon BJ, Parkinson AJ, Helminiak C, Wainwright RB, Bulkow L, Kellerman-Douglas A, et al. Response to hepatitis B vaccine of persons positive for antibody to hepatitis B core antigen. Gastroenterology 1992;103(2):590–4.
[27] Ural O, Findik D. The response of isolated anti-HBc positive subjects to recombinant hepatitis B vaccine. J Infect 2001;43(3):187–90.
[28] Murphy BL, Maynard JE, Le Bouvier QL. Viral subtypes and cross-protection in hepatitis B virus infections of chimpanzees. Intervirology 1974;3(5–6):378–81.
[29] Szmuness W, Stevens CE, Harley EJ, Zang EA, Alter HJ, Taylor PE, et al. Hepatitis B vaccine in medical staff of hemodialysis units: efficacy and subtype cross-protection. N Engl J Med 1982;307(24):1481–6.
[30] West DJ, Rabalais OP, Watson B, Keyserling HL, Matthews H, Hesley TM. Antibody responses of healthy infants to concurrent administration of a bivalent haemophilus influenzae type b-hepatitis B vaccine with diphtheria-tetanus-pertussis, polio and measles-mumps-rubella vaccines. BioDrugs 2001;15(6):413–8.
[31] Koff RS. Immunogenicity of hepatitis B vaccines: implications of immune memory. Vaccine 2002;20(31–32):3695–701.
[32] Treadwell TL, Keeffe EB, Lake J, Read A, Friedman LS, Goldman IS, et al. Immunogenicity of two recombinant hepatitis B vaccines in older individuals. Am J Med 1993;95(6): 584–8.
[33] Averhoff F, Mahoney F, Coleman P, Schatz G, Hurwitz E, Margolis H. Immunogenicity of hepatitis B Vaccines. Implications for persons at occupational risk of hepatitis B virus infection. Am J Prev Med 1998;15(1):1–8.

[34] Pillot J, Poynard T, Elias A, Maillard J, Lazizi Y, Brancer M, et al. Weak immunogenicity of the preS2 sequence and lack of circumventing effect on the unresponsiveness to the hepatitis B virus vaccine. Vaccine 1995;13(3):289–94.
[35] Clements ML, Miskovsky E, Davidson M, Cupps T, Kumwenda N, Sandman LA, et al. Effect of age on the immunogenicity of yeast recombinant hepatitis B vaccines containing surface antigen (S) or PreS2 + S antigens. J Infect Dis 1994;170(3):510–6.
[36] Weber DJ, Rutala WA, Samsa GP, Santimaw JE, Lemon SM. Obesity as a predictor of poor antibody response to hepatitis B plasma vaccine. JAMA 1985;254(22):3187–9.
[37] Shaw FE Jr, Guess HA, Roets JM, Mohr FE, Coleman PJ, Mandel EJ, et al. Effect of anatomic injection site, age and smoking on the immune response to hepatitis B vaccination. Vaccine 1989;7(5):425–30.
[38] Coleman PJ, Shaw FE Jr, Serovich J, Hadler SC, Margolis HS. Intradermal hepatitis B vaccination in a large hospital employee population. Vaccine 1991;9(10):723–7.
[39] McKinney WP, Russler SK, Horowitz MM, Battiola RJ, Lee MB. Duration of response to intramuscular versus low dose intradermal hepatitis B booster immunization. Infect Contral Hosp Epidemiol 1991;12(4):226–30.
[40] Carlsson T, Struve J, Sonnerborg A, Weiland O. The anti-HBs response after 2 different accelerated intradermal and intramuscular schemes for hepatitis B vaccination. Scand J Infect Dis 1999;31(1):93–5.
[41] Rahman F, Dahmen A, Herzog-Hauff S, Bocher WO, Galle PR, Lohr HF. Cellular and humoral immune responses induced by intradermal or intramuscular vaccination with the major hepatitis B surface antigen. Hepatology 2000;31(2):521–7.
[42] Redfield RR, Innis BL, Scott RM, Cannon HG, Bancroft WH. Clinical evaluation of low-dose intradermally administered hepatitis B virus vaccine. A cost reduction strategy. JAMA 1985;254(22):3203–6.
[43] Cardell K, Fryden A, Normann B. Intradermal hepatitis B vaccination in health care workers. Response rate and experiences from vaccination in clinical practise. Scand J Infect Dis 1999;31(2):197–200.
[44] Horowitz MM, Ershler WB, McKinney WP, Battiola RJ. Duration of immunity after hepatitis B vaccination: efficacy of low-dose booster vaccine. Ann Intern Med 1988;108(2):185–9.
[45] Wood RC, MacDonald KL, White KE, Hedberg CW, Hanson M, Osterholm MT. Risk factors for lack of detectable antibody following hepatitis B vaccination of Minnesota health care workers. JAMA 1993;270(24):2935–9.
[46] Hadler SC, de Monzon MA, Lugo DR, Perez M. Effect of timing of hepatitis B vaccine doses on response to vaccine in Yucpa Indians. Vaccine 1989;7(2):106–10.
[47] Margolis HS, Presson AC. Host factors related to poor immunogenicity of hepatitis B vaccine in adults. Another reason to immunize early. JAMA 1993;270(24):2971–2.
[48] Roome AJ, Walsh SJ, Cartter ML, Hadler JL. Hepatitis B vaccine responsiveness in Connecticut public safety personnel. JAMA 1993;270(24):2931–4.
[49] Winter AP, Follett EA, McIntyre J, Stewart J, Symington IS. Influence of smoking on immunological responses to hepatitis B vaccine. Vaccine 1994;12(9):771–2.
[50] Collier AC, Corey L, Murphy VL, Handsfield HH. Antibody to human immunodeficiency virus (HIV) and suboptimal response to hepatitis B vaccination. Ann Intern Med 1988;109(2):101–5.
[51] Hollinger FB. Factors influencing the immune response to hepatitis B vaccine, booster dose guidelines, and vaccine protocol recommendations. Am J Med 1989;87(3A):36S–40S.
[52] Craven DE, Awdeh ZL, Kunches LM, Yunis EJ, Dienstag JL, Werner BG, et al. Nonresponsiveness to hepatitis B vaccine in health care workers. Results of revaccination and genetic typings. Ann Intern Med 1986;105(3):356–60.
[53] Alper CA, Kruskall MS, Marcus-Bagley D, Craven DE, Katz AJ, Brink SJ, et al. Genetic prediction of nonresponse to hepatitis B vaccine. N Engl J Med 1989;321(11):708–12.

[54] Francis DP, Hadler SC, Thompson SE, Maynard JE, Ostrow DG, Altman N, et al. The prevention of hepatitis B with vaccine. Report of the centers for disease control multi-center efficacy trial among homosexual men. Ann Intern Med 1982;97(3):362–6.
[55] Szmuness W, Stevens CE, Harley EJ, Zang EA, Oleszko WR, William DC, et al. Hepatitis B vaccine: demonstration of efficacy in a controlled clinical trial in a high-risk population in the United States. N Engl J Med 1980;303(15):833–41.
[56] Szmuness W, Stevens CE, Zang EA, Harley EJ, Kellner A. A controlled clinical trial of the efficacy of the hepatitis B vaccine (Heptavax B): a final report. Hepatology 1981;1(5): 377–85.
[57] Wainwright RB, McMahon BJ, Bulkow LR, Hall DB, Fitzgerald MA, Harpster AP, et al. Duration of immunogenicity and efficacy of hepatitis B vaccine in a Yupik Eskimo population. JAMA 1989;261(16):2362–6.
[58] Wainwright RB, Bulkow LR, Parkinson AJ, Zanis C, McMahon BJ. Protection provided by hepatitis B vaccine in a Yupik Eskimo population—results of a 10-year study. J Infect Dis 1997;175(3):674–7.
[59] Bulkow LR, Wainwright RB, McMahon BJ, Parkinson AJ. Increases in levels of antibody to hepatitis B surface antigen in an immunized population. Clin Infect Dis 1998;26(4): 933–7.
[60] Hadler SC, Francis DP, Maynard JE, Thompson SE, Judson FN, Echenberg DF, et al. Long-term immunogenicity and efficacy of hepatitis B vaccine in homosexual men. N Engl J Med 1986;315(4):209–14.
[61] Marsano LS, West DJ, Chan I, Hesley TM, Cox J, Hackworth V, et al. A two-dose hepatitis B vaccine regimen: proof of priming and memory responses in young adults. Vaccine 1998; 16(6):624–9.
[62] Jilg W, Schmidt M, Deinhardt F. Vaccination against hepatitis B: comparison of three different vaccination schedules. J Infect Dis 1989;160(5):766–9.
[63] Szmuness W, Stevens CE, Harley EJ, Zang EA, Taylor PE, Alter HJ. The immune response of healthy adults to a reduced dose of hepatitis B vaccine. J Med Viral 1981;8(2):123–9.
[64] Stevens CE, Alter HJ, Taylor PE, Zang EA, Harley EJ, Szmuness W. Hepatitis B vaccine in patients receiving hemodialysis. Immunogenicity and efficacy. N Engl J Med 1984;311(8): 496–501.
[65] Villeneuve E, Vincelette J, Villeneuve JP. Ineffectiveness of hepatitis B vaccination in cirrhotic patients waiting for liver transplantation. Can J Gastroenterol 2000;14(Suppl B): 59B–62B.
[66] Dominguez M, Barcena R, Garcia M, Lopez-Sanroman A, Nuno J. Vaccination against hepatitis B virus in cirrhotic patients on liver transplant waiting list. Liver Transpl 2000; 6(4):440–2.
[67] Keyserling HL, West DJ, Hesley TM, Bosley C, Wiens BL, Calandra GB. Antibody responses of healthy infants to a recombinant hepatitis B vaccine administered at two, four, and twelve or fifteen months of age. J Pediatr 1994;125(1):67–9.
[68] Euler GL, Copeland JR, Rangel MC, Williams WW. Antibody response to postexposure pro-phylaxis in infants born to hepatitis B surface antigen-positive women. Pediatr Infect Dis J 2003;22(2):123–9.
[69] Prozesky OW, Stevens CE, Szmuness W, Rolka H, Harley EJ, Kew MC, et al. Immune response to hepatitis B vaccine in newboms. J Infect 1983 Jul;7(Suppl 1):53–5.
[70] West DJ, Watson B, Lichtman J, Hesley TM, Hedberg K. Persistence of immunologic memory for twelve years in children given hepatitis B vaccine in infancy. Pediatr Infect Dis J 1994;13(8):745–7.
[71] Seto D, West DJ, Ioli VA. Persistence of antibody and immunologic memory in children immunized with hepatitis B vaccine at birth. Pediatr Infect Dis J 2002;21(8):793–5.
[72] Whittle HC, Maine N, Pilkington J, Mendy M, Fortuin M, Bunn J, et al. Long-term efficacy of continuing hepatitis B vaccination in infancy in two Gambian villages. Lancet 1995; 345(8957):1089–92.

[73] Williams IT, Goldstein ST, Tufa J, Tauillii S, Margolis HS, Mahoney FJ. Long term antibody response to hepatitis B vaccination beginning at birth and to subsequent booster vaccination. Pediatr Infect Dis J 2003;22(2):157–63.
[74] Marion SA, Tomm Pastore M, Pi DW, Mathias RG. Long-term follow-up of hepatitis B vaccine in infants of carrier mothers. Am J Epidemiol 1994;140:734–6.
[75] Poovorawan Y, Chongsrisawat V, Theamboonlers A, Vimolkej L, Yano M. Is there evidence for intrauterine HBV infection in newborns of hepatitis B carrier mothers? Southeast Asian J Trop Med Public Health 1997;28(2):365–9.
[76] Lin HH, Ohto H, Etoh T, Yoneyama T, Kawana T, Mizuno M. Studies on the risk factors of intrauterine infection of hepatitis B virus. Nippon Sanka Fujinka Gakkai Zasshi 1985; 37(11):2393–400.
[77] Ohto H, Lin HH, Kawana T, Etoh T, Tohyama H. Intrauterine transmission of hepatitis B virus is closely related to placental leakage. J Med Virol 1987;21(1):1–6.
[78] Hsu HY, Chang MH, Ni YH, Lin HH, Wang SM, Chen DS. Surface gene mutants of hepatitis B virus in infants who develop acute or chronic infections despite immunoprophylaxis. Hepatology 1997;26(3):786–91.
[79] Okamoto H, Yano K, Nozaki Y, Matsui A, Miyazaki H, Yamamoto K, et al. Mutations within the S gene of hepatitis B virus transmitted from mothers to babies immunized with hepatitis B immune globulin and vaccine. Pediatr Res 1992;32(3):264–8.
[80] Zhu Q, Lu Q, Xiong S, Yu H, Duan S. Hepatitis B virus S gene mutants in infants infected despite immunoprophylaxis. Chin Med J 2001;114(4):352–4.
[81] Ni YH, Chang MH, Huang LM, Chen HL, Hsu HY, Chiu TY, et al. Hepatitis B virus infection in children and adolescents in a hyperendemic area: 15 years after mass hepatitis B vaccination. Ann Intern Med 2001;135(9):796–800.
[82] Chang MH, Chen CJ, Lai MS, Hsu HM, Wu TC, Kong MS, et al. Universal hepatitis B vaccination in Taiwan and the incidence of hepatocellular carcinoma in children. Taiwan Childhood Hepatoma Study Group. N Engl J Med 1997;336(26):1855–9.
[83] Hsu HY, Chang MH, Liaw SH, Ni YH, Chen HL. Changes of hepatitis B surface antigen variants in carrier children before and after universal vaccination in Taiwan. Hepatology 1999;30(5):1312–7.
[84] Yusuf H, Daniels D, Mast EE, Coronado V. Hepatitis B vaccination coverage among United States children. Pediatr Infect Dis J 2001;20(11 Suppl):S30–3.
[85] Struve J, Aronsson B, Frenning B, Forsgren M, Weiland O. Seroconversion after additional vaccine doses to non-responders to three doses of intradermally or intramuscularly administered recombinant hepatitis B vaccine. Scand J Infect Dis 1994;26(4): 468–70.
[86] Sjogren MH. Prevention of hepatitis B in nonresponders to initial hepatitis B vaccination. Am J Med 2005;118:34S–9S.
[87] Bertino JS Jr, Tirrell P, Greenberg RN, Keyserling HL, Poland GA, Gump D, et al. A comparative trial of standard or high-dose S subunit recombinant hepatitis B vaccine versus a vaccine containing S subunit, pre-S1, and pre-S2 particles for revaccination of healthy adult nonresponders. J Infect Dis 1997;175(3):678–81.
[88] Goldwater PN. Randomized, comparative trial of 20 micrograms vs 40 micrograms Engerix B vaccine in hepatitis B vaccine non-responders. Vaccine 1997;15(4):353–6.
[89] Gupta RK, Relyveld EH, Lindblad EB, Bizzini B, Ben-Efraim S, Gupta CK. Adjuvants—a balance between toxicity and adjuvanticity. Vaccine 1993;11(3):293–306.
[90] Lin R, Tarr PE, Jones TC. Present status of the use of cytokines as adjuvants with vaccines to protect against infectious diseases. Clin Infect Dis 1995;21(6):1439–49.
[91] Jones T, Stem A, Lin R. Potential role of granulocyte-macrophage colony-stimulating factor as vaccine adjuvant. Eur J Clin Microbiol Infect Dis 1994;13(Suppl 2): S47–53.
[92] Taglietti M. Vaccine adjuvancy: a new potential area of development for GM-CSF. Adv Exp Med Biol 1995;378:565–9.

[93] Kim MJ, Nafziger AN, Harro CD, Keyserling HL, Ramsey KM, Drusano GL, et al. Revaccination of healthy nonrespondere with hepatitis B vaccine and prediction of seroprotection response. Vaccine 2003;21(11–12):1174–9.
[94] Vlassopoulos D. Recombinant hepatitis B vaccination in renal failure patients. Curr Pharm Biotechnol 2003;4(2):141–51.
[95] Kovacic V, Sain M, Vukman V. Efficient haemodialysis improves the response to hepatitis B virus vaccination. Intervirology 2002;45(3):172–6.
[96] Sudhagar K, Chandrasekar S, Rao MS, Ravichandran R. Effect of granulocyte macrophage colony stimulating factor on hepatitis-B vaccination in haemodialysis patients. J Assoc Physicians India 1999;47(6):602–4.
[97] Singh NP, Mandal SK, Thakur A, Kapoor D, Anuradha S, Prakash A, et al. Efficacy of GM-CSF as an adjuvant to hepatitis B vaccination in patients with chronic renal failure—results of a prospective, randomized trial. Ren Fail 2003;25(2):255–66.
[98] Anandh U, Bastani B, Ballal S. Granulocyte-macrophage colony-stimulating factor as an adjuvant to hepatitis B vaccination in maintenance hemodialysis patients. Am J Nephrol 2000;20(1):53–6.
[99] Jha R, Lakhtakia S, Jaleel MA, Narayan G, Hemlatha K. Granulocyte macrophage colony stimulating factor (GM-CSF) induced sero-protection in end stage renal failure patients to hepatitis B in vaccine non-responders. Ren Fail 2001;23(5):629–36.
[100] Evans TG, Schiff M, Graves B, Agosti J, Barritt ML, Garner D, et al. The safety and efficacy of GM-CSF as an adjuvant in hepatitis B vaccination of chronic hemodialysis patients who have failed primary vaccination. Clin Nephrol 2000;54(2):138–42.
[101] Hess G, Kreiter F, Kosters W, Deusch K. The effect of granulocyte-macrophage colony-stimulating factor (GM-CSF) on hepatitis B vaccination in haemodialysis patients. J Viral Hepat 1996;3(3):149–53.
[102] Stratton KR, Howe CJ, Johnston RB Jr. Adverse events associated with childhood vaccines other than pertussis and rubella: summary of a report from the Institute of Medicine. JAMA 1994;271:1602–5.
[103] McMahon BJ, Helminiak C, Wainwright RB, Bulkow L, Trimble BA, Wainwright K. Frequency of adverse reactions to hepatitis B vaccine in 43,618 persons. Am J Med 1992;92(3): 254–6.
[104] Shaw FE Jr, Graham DJ, Guess HA, Milstien JB, Johnson JM, Schatz GC, et al. Postmarketing surveillance for neurologic adverse events reported after hepatitis B vaccination. Experience of the first three years. Am J Epidemiol 1988;127(2):337–52.
[105] Ascherio A, Zhang SM, Hernan MA, Olek MJ, Coplan PM, Brodovicz K, et al. Hepatitis B vaccination and the risk of multiple sclerosis. N Engl J Med 2001;344(5):327–32.
[106] Pol S, Nalpas B, Driss F, Michel ML, Tiollais P, Denis J, et al. Efficacy and limitations of a specific immunotherapy in chronic hepatitis B. J Hepatol 2001;34(6):917–21.

ELSEVIER
SAUNDERS

Infect Dis Clin N Am
20 (2006) 47–61

INFECTIOUS
DISEASE CLINICS
OF NORTH AMERICA

Serologic and Molecular Diagnosis of Hepatitis B Virus

Julie C. Servoss, MD[a,b],
Lawrence S. Friedman, MD[a,c,d,*]

[a]Department of Medicine, Harvard Medical School, Boston, MA 02114, USA
[b]Gastrointestinal Unit, Blake 4, Massachusetts General Hospital, 55 Fruit Street, Boston, MA 02114, USA
[c]Department of Medicine, Newton-Wellesley Hospital, 2014 Washington Street, Newton, MA 02462, USA
[d]Department of Medicine, Massachusetts General Hospital, Boston, MA 02114, USA

Hepatitis B virus (HBV) is a hepadnavirus with a 3200-base-pair genome that consists of partially double-stranded DNA (dsDNA) and a lipoprotein outer envelope (Fig. 1). The HBV genome has four overlapping open reading frames with four major genes designated pre-S/S, C, P, and X. The pre-S genes (S1 and S2) code for the hepatocyte receptor–binding site, whereas the S (surface) gene codes for hepatitis B surface antigen (HBsAg). The C (core) gene codes for hepatitis B core antigen (HBcAg) and hepatitis B e antigen (HBeAg), whereas the P (polymerase) gene encodes the HBV DNA polymerase. The X gene encodes a protein that transactivates transcriptional promoters. Eight genotypes (A–H) of HBV have been identified based on nucleotide sequence divergences of at least 8%. HBV genotypes differ in their predominant geographic occurrence and response to therapy with interferon. Genotype A is the predominant genotype in the United States and is more responsive to interferon than genotype D which predominates in the Middle East and South Asia [1].

After a person is exposed to the virus, the serologic course of HBV infection begins approximately 6 to 10 weeks after exposure with the appearance of HBsAg and HBeAg, a marker of active HBV replication. (HBV DNA may be detectable in serum up to 21 days before the appearance of HBsAg

A version of this article originally appeared in the 8:2 issue of Clinics in Liver Disease.

* Corresponding author. Department of Medicine, Newton-Wellesley Hospital, 2014 Washington Street, Newton, MA 02462.

E-mail address: lfriedman@partners.org (L.S. Friedman).

0891-5520/06/$ - see front matter
doi:10.1016/j.idc.2006.01.005

id.theclinics.com

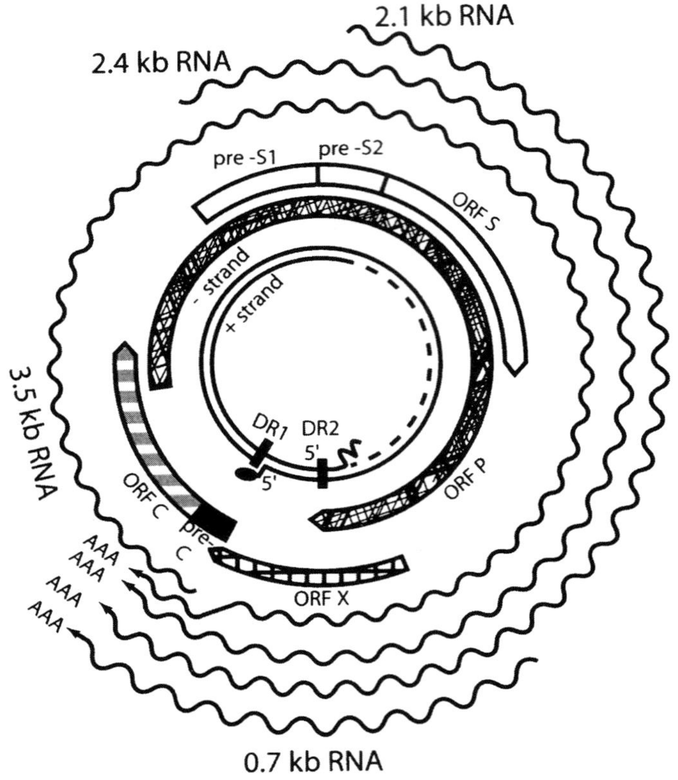

Fig. 1. Genomic organization of HBV Partially double-stranded DNA (complete minus strand and partial plus strand); the major viral mRNA coded by these regions (wavy lines on the outer circle); and resultant proteins (S, P, C, and X) from the four open reading frames (ORF). The filled circle at the 5′ end of the minus strand DNA represents the terminal protein; the wavy line at the 5′ end of the plus strand denotes the terminal RNA. DR1 and DR2 are the direct repeats, which are important for the initiation of viral DNA synthesis. (*From* Ganem D. Hepadnaviridae: the viruses and their replication. In: Fields BN, Knipe DM, Hawley PM, editors. Fundamental virology. 3rd edition. Philadelphia: Lippincott-Raven; 1996. p. 1199–234; with permission.)

[Fig. 2]). Patients then exhibit increased serum aminotransferase levels, usually $\geq$ 500 U/L, with the serum alanine aminotransferase (ALT) typically higher than the aspartate aminotransferase (AST) level. Approximately 10 weeks after exposure to HBV, patients may develop nonspecific symptoms such as fatigue and malaise as well as right upper quadrant pain and jaundice. At this time, antibody to hepatitis B core antigen (anti-HBc) of the IgM class appears in the serum. In the recovery phase of HBV infection, serum aminotransferase levels return to normal, HBeAg disappears and antibody to HBeAg (anti-HBe) appears in serum, and ultimately, HBsAg seroconversion to antibody to HBsAg (anti-HBs) occurs. IgM anti-HBc

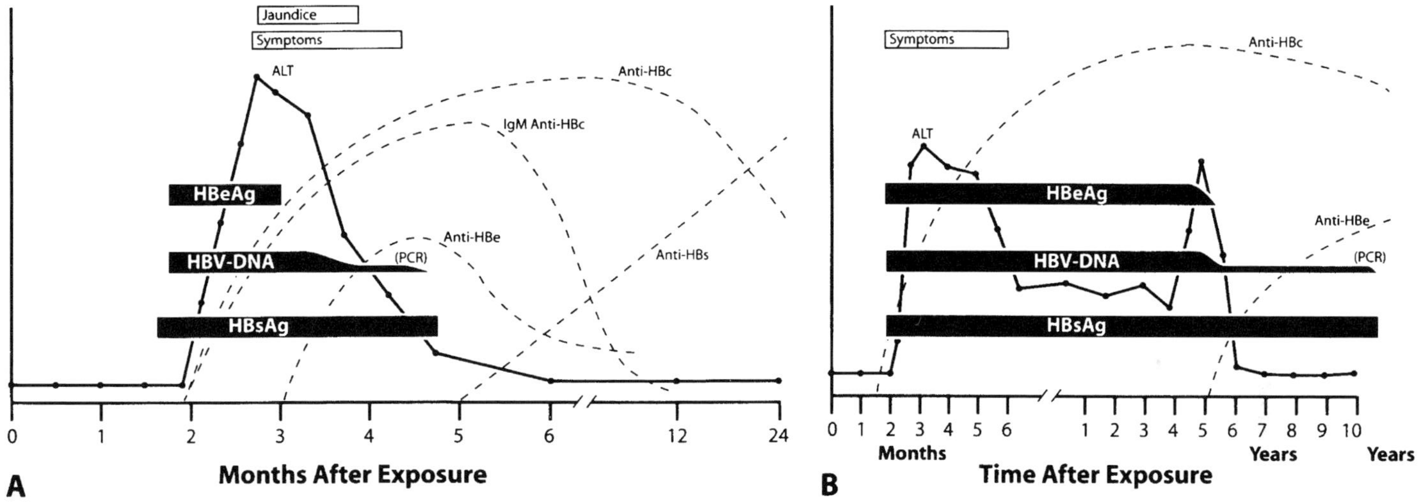

Fig. 2. Sequence of events after HBV infection. (*A*) Acute HBV infection with resolution. (*B*) Acute HBV infection progressing to chronic HBV infection. (*From* Hoofnagle JH, DiBisceglie AM. Serologic diagnosis of acute and chronic viral hepatitis. Semin Liver Dis 1991;11:73–83; with permission.)

levels begin to decline as levels of anti-HBc of the IgG class rise in serum. Recovery from acute HBV infection is typically associated with undetectable serum levels of HBV DNA. However, using polymerase chain reaction (PCR) techniques (see later discussion), low levels (10^1 to 10^2 genome equivalents/mL) of HBV DNA have been found in serum and peripheral blood mononuclear cells of patients up to 21 years after clinical and serologic recovery from HBV infection [2].

The hallmark of progression to chronic HBV infection is the presence of HBsAg for more than 6 months. Typically, in the early, or replicative, phase of chronic HBV infection, markers of active viral replication, HBeAg and serum HBV DNA levels $> 10^5$ copies/mL, are present. Patients may ultimately enter a nonreplicative state characterized by seroconversion from HBeAg to anti-HBe, serum HBV DNA levels $< 10^5$ copies/mL, and normalization of serum aminotransferase levels. This phase is also referred to as the inactive carrier state. It is important to note that up to 20% of patients in the inactive carrier state may experience a reactivation to the replicative state, or flare, and may even cycle between the nonreplicative and replicative state [3]. Such flares are characterized by an increase in serum aminotransferase levels and serum HBV DNA levels to $> 10^5$ copies/mL, with or without seroreversion to HBeAg. Reappearance of HBeAg may or may not occur during reactivation (see later discussion).

Several clinically important mutations in the HBV genome have been described. A subset of patients with chronic HBV infection has HBeAg-negative chronic hepatitis B characterized by circulating HBV DNA, fluctuating serum aminotransferase levels, and, in some cases, severe hepatic necroinflammatory activity and even liver failure. This occurs as a result of mutations in the precore or core region of HBV DNA. The most common precore mutation is a single amino acid substitution of adenosine (A) for guanine (G) at nucleotide position 1896 ($G_{1896}A$) that results in a premature stop codon that inhibits the production of HBeAg [4]. The most common core mutations include single amino acid substitutions of threonine (T) for adenosine (A) at position 1762 ($A_{1762}T$) and adenosine (A) for guanine (G) at position 1764 ($G_{1764}A$) that result in decreased translation of HBeAg. These core promoter variants have been associated with 10% of cases of fulminant HBV infection and 27% of cases of progressive chronic hepatitis B (see also chapter in this issue by Drs. Wai and Fontana [5].

Other important mutations occur in the YMDD (tyrosine-methionine-aspar-tate-aspartate) motif of the DNA polymerase gene and include substitutions of valine (V) for methionine (M) ($M_{204}V$), isoleucine (I) for methionine ($M_{204}I$), or methionine for leucine (L) ($L_{180}M$). These mutations occur during treatment of chronic hepatitis B infection with lamivudine, a nucleoside analogue, and result in the formation of bulky side chains that inhibit the binding of lamivudine. The emergence of these lamivudine-resistant mutants may be accompanied by HBeAg to anti-HBe seroconversion, a flare of serum aminotransferase levels, or hepatic decompensation. Mutations that lead to resistance occur less frequently during the course of therapy with other nucleoside or nucleotide analogs, such as adefovir, entecavir, and tenofovir [6].

Serologic diagnosis of hepatitis B virus

Serologic diagnosis of HBV can be accomplished by identifying virally encoded antigens and their corresponding antibodies: HBsAg, anti-HBs, HBeAg, anti-HBe, and anti-HBc. (HBcAg does not circulate freely in the serum [Table 1].)

Acute hepatitis B virus infection

HBsAg, a product of the S gene, is part of the surface envelope of HBV and also circulates in excess ($\sim 10^{13}$ particles/mL) in the serum as non-virion associated spheres and tubules [7]. HBsAg is the first marker of acute HBV infection and appears as early as 1 week after initial exposure to HBV and before the onset of symptoms or serum aminotransferase elevations (see Fig. 2). Typically, HBsAg becomes detectable by 6 to 10 weeks after exposure to the virus. In acute, resolving HBV infection, serum HBsAg levels begin to fall 4 to 6 months after exposure, as anti-HBs levels increase. For most patients, the presence of anti-HBs heralds resolving HBV infection and subsequent lifelong immunity. HBsAg and anti-HBs can be detected in

Table 1
Interpretation of serologic and molecular markers of hepatitis B virus during different stages of infection

Stage of HBV infection	HBsAg	Anti-HBs	HBeAg	Anti-HBe	Anti-HBc	HBV DNA
Acute HBV infection						
Early	+	−	+	−	IgM	+
Window period	−	−	−	−	IgM	+/−
Recovery	−	+	−	+	IgG	+/−[a]
Chronic HBV infection						
Replicative	+	−	+	−	IgG, IgM[b]	$>10^5$ copies/mL
Nonreplicative/inactive carrier state	+	−	−	+	IgG	$<10^5$ copies/mL
Reactivation HBV	+	−	+/−	−	IgM	$>10^5$ copies/mL
HBeAg(-) chronic HBV (precore or core mutant)	+	−	−	+	IgG	$>10^5$ copies/mL

Abbreviations: anti-HBc, antibody to hepatitis B core antigen; anti-HBe, antibody to hepatitis B e antigen; anti-HBs, antibody to hepatitis B surface antigen; HBeAg, hepatitis B e antigen; HBsAg, hepatitis B surface antigen; HBV, hepatitis B virus; IgG, IgG class of antibody; IgM, IgM class of antibody.

[a] Low levels (10^1–10^2 genome equivalents/mL) may be detected in serum up to 21 years after recovery from acute HBV infection.

[b] Low levels may also be detected.

the serum using enzyme immunoassays (EIAs). The positive predictive value of the assay for predicting an anti-HBs titer $\geq$ 10 mIU/mL, which is associated with immunity, is 97.6% [8].

When less sensitive assays for HBsAg and anti-HBs were used in the past, patients with acute HBV infection were often noted to have a window period during which neither HBsAg nor anti-HBs was detectable in the serum (see Fig. 2); with contemporary assays, this window period is rarely, if ever, observed [9]. During the window period, the presence of IgM anti-HBc was used to diagnose acute HBV infection. IgM anti-HBc is still a reliable marker of acute hepatitis B but may also be detected during flares of chronic hepatitis B (see later discussion). HBcAg, a component of the nucleocapsid protein, is associated with the intact virion and does not circulate freely in the serum; therefore, HBcAg cannot be detected by standard assays. During acute or recent HBV infection, IgM anti-HBc appears shortly after HBsAg and persists for 6 to 24 months after exposure to HBV. During the course of acute HBV infection, IgG anti-HBc appears and eventually replaces IgM anti-HBc. The presence of IgG anti-HBc signifies either resolved HBV infection (when detected with anti-HBs after clearance of HBsAg) or chronic HBV infection (when detected in patients with persistent HBsAg). There are commercially available EIAs for total anti-HBc and IgM anti-HBc. The presence of IgG anti-HBc is inferred when total anti-HBc is present but levels of IgM anti-HBc are undetectable.

Occasionally, people are found to have an isolated anti-HBc in the absence of HBsAg or anti-HBs. For example, up to 5% of healthy blood donors have isolated anti-HBc in the serum. Among human immunodeficiency virus (HIV)–infected people, the rate of isolated anti-HBc in serum is as high as 42% [10]. Isolated anti-HBc can occur in four settings: (1) during the window period of acute HBV infection (see earlier discussion); (2) during chronic HBV infection as levels of HBsAg become undetectable; (3) after resolved HBV infection in the remote past as anti-HBs levels fall below the limits of detection; and (4) as a false-positive result. Up to 20% of people with isolated anti-HBc in serum have circulating HBV DNA, signifying chronic HBV infection [11–13]. In the other 80% of cases, the isolated anti-HBc usually represents a false-positive result or HBV infection in the remote past. It is important to test for low levels of HBV DNA by molecular assays in patients with isolated anti-HBc to identify occult chronic HBV infection (see later discussion).

HBeAg is almost invariably detected during acute HBV infection, in which case HBsAg and IgM anti-HBc are also usually present. During the course of chronic HBV infection, detection of HBeAg generally signifies active viral replication and infectivity. HBeAg is translated from the C gene of HBV. Unlike HBcAg, HBeAg is released in the serum and can be detected in the serum by EIA. In the course of acute HBV infection, HBeAg is detectable between 6 and 12 weeks after exposure to HBV. For patients who successfully clear the virus from serum, HBeAg levels decline with seroconversion to anti-HBe in association with a marked decline in HBV DNA levels in serum. Persistence of HBeAg in serum beyond the first 3 or 4 months of acute HBV infection usually portends development of chronic HBV infection.

Chronic hepatitis B virus infection

Chronic HBV infection is diagnosed by the presence of HBsAg for more than 6 months, serum HBV DNA > 10^5 copies/mL, and persistent or intermittent elevations of serum ALT or AST levels [14]. Chronic HBV infection can be further divided into HBeAg-positive and HBeAg-negative chronic HBV infection. The typical patient with chronic HBV infection has both HBsAg and HBeAg in serum, reflecting active viral replication, infectivity, and hepatic inflammation.

Three epidemiologic patterns of HBeAg-positive chronic HBV infection, defined by mode of transmission, have been identified. Pattern 1 is typical of chronic HBV infection resulting from perinatal transmission, in which HBeAg seroconversion usually does not occur until adulthood [3], This pattern is seen predominantly in Asia and Oceania, where patients present with HBeAg positivity, high serum HBV DNA levels, and normal serum aminotransferase levels, reflecting an "immune tolerant" state [3]. People with Pattern 1 chronic HBV infection may episodically exhibit elevated serum aminotransferase levels and other evidence of ongoing liver injury.

Pattern 2 chronic HBV infection is seen primarily in sub-Saharan Africa, Alaska, and Mediterranean countries where people become infected with HBV during childhood through person-to-person contact [3]. Typically, these people have HBeAg in serum, elevated serum HBV DNA levels, and elevated serum aminotransferase levels. During the course of infection, seroconversion from HBeAg to anti-HBe may occur, often around puberty.

Pattern 3 chronic HBV infection, which is most common in the United States, occurs among people who are infected with HBV through sexual transmission [3]. As with pattern 2, affected people tend to have HBeAg in serum, elevated serum HBV DNA levels, and elevated serum AST or ALT levels (Fig. 2). These findings indicate active hepatic necroinflammation.

Most people with HBeAg-positive chronic HBV infection who undergo seroconversion to anti-HBe will subsequently have sustained control of the HBV infection, with normal serum aminotransferase levels and low (< 10^5 copies/mL) or undetectable serum levels of HBV DNA, although HBsAg remains detectable in serum. These people are known as inactive carriers. However, some people who are HBeAg-negative and anti-HBe-positive still have active chronic HBV infection. Despite the of circulating HBeAg. suchjeopjejiave detectable HBV DNA (> 10^5 copies/mL) and fluctuating serum ALT or AS levels [14]. The lack of HBeAg occurs as a result of precore or core promoter region mutations in the HBV DNA that halt production of HBeAg. As discussed earlier, the most commonly seen precore mutation is the $G_{1896}A$ substitution that results in a stop codon. This HBV mutant can be found in 10% to 15% of people with chronic HBV infection in the United States and Europe and 40% to 80% of people with chronic HBV infection in Southern Europe, the Middle East, and Asia [15]. When compared with people with HBeAg-positive chronic HBV infection, the clinical course of people with HBeAg-negative chronic HBV infection typically is characterized by lower serum HBV DNA levels and intermittent, rather than sustained, periods of necroinflammatory activity in the liver. In addition, long-term antiviral therapy is generally required to maintain suppression of HBV replication.

Treatment of HBeAg-positive or HBeAg-negative chronic HBV infection with lamivudine, a nucleoside analogue, is complicated by the development of lamivudine-resistant HBV mutants, specifically mutations in the YMDD (tyrosine-methionine-aspartate-aspartate) motif of the HBV DNA polymerase gene. These mutations occur in 17% of patients at 1 year of treatment with lamivudine, 40% at 2 years, 55% at 3 years, and 67% at 4 years [14]. A commercially available PCR test (Hepatitis B Virus GenotypR, Roche Molecular Systems, Specialty Laboratories, Santa Monica, California) is available to identify the most common mutations in the DNA polymerase gene: $M_{552}V$, $M_{552}I$, or $L_{528}M$.

Molecular diagnosis of hepatitis B virus

Clinical applications of hepatitis B virus DNA assays

The diagnosis of acute and chronic HBV infection can be made using the serologic tests described previously. However, the ability to perform quantitative tests in serum for HBV DNA is useful in several settings: (1) to diagnose some cases of acute HBV infection; (2) to distinguish replicative from non-replicative chronic HBV infection; and (3) to monitor a patient's response to antiviral therapy. Determination of the HBV genotype will likely be used in the future to help predict response to antiviral therapy and can be performed with a commercially available line probe assay (INNO-LiPA HBV Genotyping Assay, Immunogenetics N.V., Ghent, Belgium) [16].

In most instances, the diagnosis of acute hepatitis B can be made with serologic testing for HBsAg. Coincident with the appearance of HBsAg in serum, markers of active HBV replication and infectivity, specifically HBeAg and HBV DNA, appear. If the results of tests for HBsAg are equivocal, assays for HBV DNA in serum may be a useful adjunct in the diagnosis of acute HBV infection. Moreover, HBV DNA can be detected approximately 21 days before HBsAg appears in the serum [17]. Thus, HBV DNA assays may be used to diagnose acute HBV infection in those patients with high-risk exposures, such as needlestick accidents in health care workers.

Assays for HBV DNA in serum are also used to characterize the replicative state of chronic HBV infection. Patients with chronic HBV infection may continue to display markers of active viral replication or may cycle between an active replicative and a nonreplicative state (see earlier discussion). Patients who cycle from a nonreplicative state to an active replicative state are said to have reactivated HBV infection. Reactivation of HBV infection may occur with or without reappearance of HBeAg in serum. With the increasing sensitivity of molecular assays that allows quantification of HBV DNA levels, the threshold that distinguishes the replicative from the nonreplicative state has been defined as 10^5 copies of HBV DNA/mL. These assays allow patients to be classified as having replicative, nonreplicative, or reactivation HBV infection. Furthermore, in patients with precore or core mutations resulting in HBeAg-negative chronic HBV infection, HBeAg cannot be relied on as a marker of active viral replication, and detection of HBV DNA is necessary for confirmation of an active replicative state.

In addition to characterizing the status of viral replication in patients with chronic HBV infection, quantitative HBV DNA assays are useful in monitoring response to antiviral treatment. Recently, the National Institute of Diabetes and Digestive and Kidney Diseases and the American Gastroenterological Association proposed criteria to define response to antiviral therapy based on biochemical (BR), histologic (HR), and virologic response (VR) [14]. BR refers to a decrease in serum ALT to the normal range, and HR refers to a decrease in histologic activity index by at least 2 points compared with findings on a pretreatment liver biopsy. A critical component of VR is undetectable HBV DNA levels ($<10^5$ copies/mL) with the use of an unamplified assay (see later discussion) and loss of HBeAg in serum in patients who were initially HBeAg-positive. For patients with HBeAg-negative chronic HBV infection, however, the only measure of virologic response is loss of HBV DNA. For patients with HBV infection who are treated with lamivudine, the emergence of a lamivudine-resistant strain is characterized by the reappearance of HBV DNA in serum after an initial decline in level or disappearance.

Molecular techniques for the detection and quantification of hepatitis B virus DNA

There are both qualitative and quantitative assays for HBV DNA. However, the qualitative, PCR-based, assays are not necessary to assess the success of treatment of HBV infection, characterized by suppression of HBV DNA in serum, which can be adequately assessed by quantitative, non–PCR-based, HBV DNA assays. Quantification of HBV DNA in serum is performed using either signal or target amplification techniques. Signal amplification techniques require the use of a specific "capture" oligonucleotide probe that hybridizes to denatured DNA [17]. Then, the signal (radioisotope, chemi luminescence) from the probe-DNA hybrid is amplified for detection and quantification [17], Target amplification requires amplification of the viral genome (amplicons); the amplicons are then detected and quantified.

Assays using signal amplification include liquid hybridization (Genostics assay, Abbott Laboratories, Chicago, Illinois), the Hybrid Capture System (Digene Hybrid Capture II HBV DNA Test, Digene Corp., Gaithersburg, Maryland), and a branched DNA (bDNA) assay (Bayer, Emeryville, California). The liquid hybridization assay uses iodine 125-labeled nucleic acid probes that hybridize to soluble, denatured HBV DNA [9]. After hybridization, the radiolabeled probes are detected and quantified using a gamma scintillation counter [18]. The sensitivity of liquid hybridization is 6×10^5 copies/mL or 1–2 pg/mL [9].

In the Hybrid Capture System [17,19,20], specific RNA probes are hybridized to the target HBV DNA to create RNA–DNA hybrids (Fig. 3). Then, multiple RNA–DNA hybrids are captured onto microplate wells, using

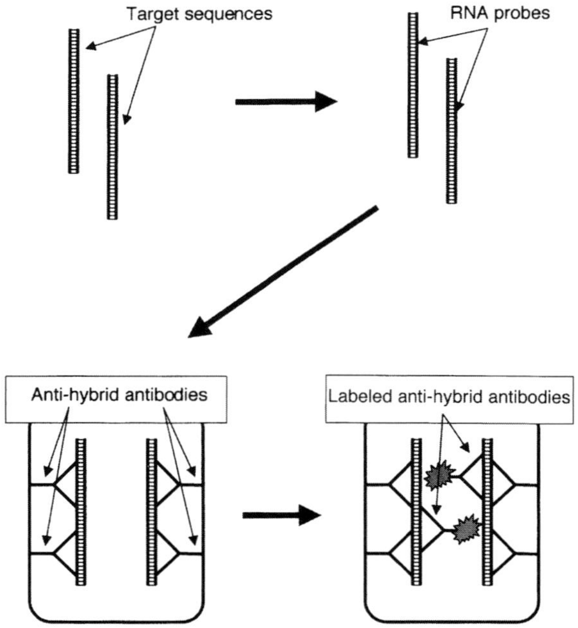

Fig. 3. Principle of hybrid capture signal amplification assay. The target sequence is double-stranded HBV DNA. Hybridization to specific RNA probes creates RNA–DNA hybrids, which are captured on a solid phase (a tube in the first-generation assay, a microplate in the second-generation assay) by means of universal capture antibodies specific for RNA–DNA hybrids. Detection is performed after signal amplification with multiple antibodies conjugated to a revelation system based on chemiluminescence. Light emission is measured and compared with a standard curve generated simultaneously with known standards. (*From* Pawlotsky J. Molecular diagnosis of viral hepatitis. Gastroenterology 2002;122:1554–68; with permission from the American Gastroenterological Association.)

universal capture antibodies specific for the hybrids. The captured RNA–DNA hybrids are then detected using multiple antibodies (creating signal amplification) conjugated to alkaline phosphatase. The bound alkaline phosphatase is detected with a chemiluminescent dioxetane substrate that produces light, which is then measured. The signal can be amplified 3000 fold. The sensitivity of the Hybrid Capture System is 4700 copies/mL [17].

The bDNA technique [17,21] involves the use of specific oligonucleotide probes to hybridize HBV DNA to plastic microwells (Fig. 4). Signal

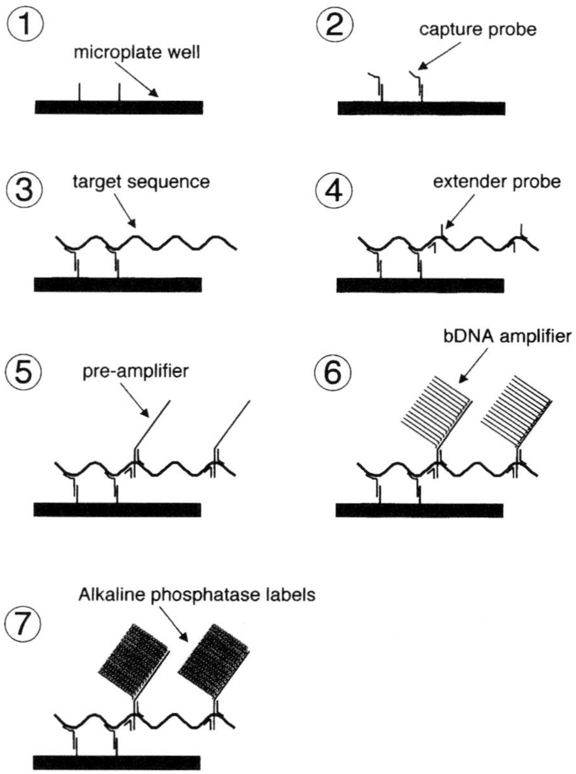

Fig. 4. Principle of branched DNA (bDNA) signal amplification assay. The target sequences are captured on the wells of a microtiter plate by means of specific "capture probes." "Extender probes" are used to hybridize synthetic bDNA amplifier molecules (in first-generation HBV DNA and hepatitis C virus (HCV) RNA assays, and in second-generation HCV RNA assays) or, as shown in the figure, preamplifier molecules that in turn hybridize bDNA molecules (third-generation HCV and HBV assays). The multiple repeat sequences within each bDNA molecule serve as sites for hybridization to alkaline phosphatase–conjugated oligonucleotide probes. Alkaline phosphatase catalyzes chemiluminescence emission from a substrate, which is measured and compared with a standard curve generated simultaneously with known standards. (*From* Pawlotsky J. Molecular diagnosis of viral hepatitis. Gastroenterology 2002;122:1554–68; with permission from the American Gastroenterological Association.)

amplification occurs when bDNA amplifier molecules are hybridized to the target HBV DNA hybrids in the microwell. Multiple repeat sequences within the bDNA amplifier molecule are then conjugated with an alkaline phosphatase–catalyzed chemiluminescence probe similar to that used in the Hybrid Capture System. The lower limit of detection for the bDNA assay is 7×10^5 DNA equivalents/mL [17].

Although the signal amplification techniques offer highly specific assays to detect HBV DNA, they are unable to detect low levels of HBV DNA ($< \sim 5{,}000$ copies/mL). Target amplification techniques such as PCR-based assays are highly sensitive with the ability to detect as few as 10 copies/mL of HBV DNA (TaqMan-based PCR) [22]. PCR assays rely on the use of specific primers that attach to each strand of target dsDNA, Then, new DNA strands are synthesized and amplified behind the primer. This cycle of DNA denaturing, primer annealing, and strand synthesis is repeated multiple times, thereby resulting in amplification of the target HBV DNA. The most common primers used in HBV DNA PCR assays are complementary to the precore or core region [9], Commercially available assays include the Amplicor HBV Monitor Test, v2.0 (Roche Molecular Systems, Pleasanton, California) and the Cobas Amplicor HBV Monitor Test, v2.0 (Roche Molecular Systems, Pleasanton, California). The ranges of HBV DNA detection are 1000 to 40,000,000 copies/mL and 200 to 200,000 copies/mL, respectively. The Cobas Amplicor system is the more sensitive of the two assays and uses an Amplicor analyzer that automates the amplification and detection process.

Recent advances in PCR technology include the development of "real-time" PCR techniques to increase the sensitivity of the assay. Real-time PCR refers to the simultaneous amplification and quantification of viral genomes, thereby obviating the need for post-PCR manipulations [23,24]. Real-time PCR can detect a wide range of HBV DNA levels and offers a more rapid assay than conventional PCR techniques. In a recent study, LightCycler (LC)-PCR (Roche Diagnostics, Pleasanton, California), a real-time PCR technique, was compared with the Hybrid Capture II HBV DNA test (Digene Corp., Gaithersburg, Maryland) [23], and LC-PCR was found to be rapid ($\sim$2.5 hours) and 500 times more sensitive than Hybrid Capture II, with an HBV DNA detection range of 250 to 2.5×10^9 copies/mL. Currently, real-time PCR using the TaqMan probe is the most sensitive quantitative HBV DNA assay and is able to detect as few as 10 copies/mL [22,25]. TaqMan technology uses a fluorescent probe annealed to target DNA sequences for quantification of DNA [26,27].

Although advances in PCR technology have permitted the detection of as few as 10 copies/mL of HBV DNA, the clinical significance of such low serum levels of HBV DNA is unknown. An arbitrary value of 10^5 copies/mL of HBV DNA has been selected as one of the diagnostic criteria for chronic HBV infection. However, this definition is problematic for several reasons. First, patients with chronic HBV infection can have HBV DNA levels that

Table 2
Commercially available hepatitis B virus DNA quantification assays

Assay	Manufacturer	Method	Lower detection cutoff	Dynamic range of quantification
Signal amplification				
Genostics Assay	Abbott Labs, Chicago, IL	Liquid hybridization	1–2 pg/mL (~600,000 copies/mL)	1–2 pg/mL –~ 800 pg/mL (600,000–300,000,000 copies/mL)
Versant HBV DNA 1.0 Assay	Bayer Corp, Diagnostics Division, Tarrytown, NY	Manual branched DNA (bDNA) signal amplification	700,000 genome equivalents/mL	700,000–5,000,000,000 genome equivalents/mL
HBV Hybrid-Capture I	Digene Corp., Gaithersburg, MD	Hybrid capture signal amplification in tubes	700,000 copies/mL	700,000–560,000,000 copies/mL
HBV Hybrid-Capture II	Digene Corp., Gaithersburg, MD	Hybrid capture signal amplification in microplates	142,000 copies/mL	142,000–1,700,000,000 copies/mL
Ultra-sensitive HBV Hybrid-Capture II	Digene Corp., Gaithersburg, MD	Hybrid capture signal amplification in microplates after centrifugation	4700 copies/rnL	4700–57,000,000 copies/mL
Target amplification				
Amplicor HBV Monitor Test v2.0	Roche Molecular Systems, Pleasanton, CA	Manual quantitative RT-PCR	1000 copies/mL	1000–40,000,000 copies/mL
Cobas Amplicor HBV Monitor Test v2.0	Roche Molecular Systems, Pleasanton, CA	Semi-automated quantitative RT-PCR	200 copies/mL	200–200,000 copies/mL

Adapted from Pawlotsky J. Molecular diagnosis of viral hepatitis. Gastroenterology 2002;122:1554–68; with permission from the American Gastroenterological Association.)

fluctuate and intermittently fall below 10^5 copies/mL. Second, the threshold HBV DNA level associated with the development of hepatic fibrosis is unknown. Third, currently available HBV DNA assays have not been standardized with respect to HBV DNA quantitative units [3] (Table 2). The World Health Organization recently established an international standard for HBV DNA assays [28]. Implementation of this standard will be essential to defining clinically appropriate treatment guidelines based on serum HBV DNA levels [17].

Summary

Serologic assays for HBV are the mainstay diagnostic tools for HBV infection. However, the advent of molecular biology–based techniques has added a new dimension to the diagnosis and treatment of patients with chronic HBV infection. Over the past decade, improvements in molecular technology, permitting detection of as few as 10 copies/mL of HBV DNA in serum have led to redefinitions of chronic HBV infection, as well as thresholds for antiviral treatment. As the sensitivity of these molecular techniques continues to improve, the challenge will be to standardize these assays as well as define clinically significant levels of HBV replication.

References

[1] Schaefer S. Hepatitis B virus: significance of genotypes. J Viral Hepat 2005;12:111–24.
[2] Cabrerizo M, Bartolome J, Caramelo C, Barril G, Carreno V. Molecular analysis of hepatitis B virus DNA in serum and peripheral blood mononuclear cells from hepatitis B surface antigen-negative cases. Hepatology 2000;32:116–23.
[3] Lok ASF, McMahon BJ. Chronic hepatitis B. Hepatology 2001;34:1225–41.
[4] Okamoto H, Tsuda F, Akahane Y, Sugai Y, Toshiba M, Moriyama K, et al. Hepatitis B virus with mutations in the core promoter for an e antigen-negative phenotype in carriers with antibody to e antigen. J Virol 1994;68:8102–10.
[5] Laskus T, Rakela J, Nowicki MJ, Pershing DH. Hepatitis B core promoter sequence analysis in fulminant and chronic hepatitis B. Gastroenterology 1995;109:1618–23.
[6] Locarnini S. Molecular virology and the development of resistant mutants: implications for therapy. Semin Liver Dis 2005;25(Suppl 1):9–19.
[7] Martin P, Friedman LS, Dienstag JL. Diagnostic approach. In: Zuckerman AJ, Thomas HC, editors. Viral hepatitis: scientific basis and clinical management. Edinburgh: Churchill Living-stone; 1993. p. 393–408.
[8] CDC. Sensitivity of the test for antibody to hepatitis B surface antigen—United States. MMWR 1993;42:707–10.
[9] Berenguer M, Wright TL. Viral hepatitis. In: Feldman M, Friedman LS, Sleisenger MH, editors. Sleisenger and Fordtran's gastrointestinal and liver disease: pathophysiology diagnosis management. 7th edition. Philadelphia: W.B. Saunders; 2002. p. 1278–341.
[10] Gandhi RT, Wurcel A, Lee H, McGovern B, Boczanowski M, Gerwin R, et al. Isolated antibody to hepatitis B core antigen in human immunodeficiency virus type-1–infected individuals. Clin Infect Dis 2003;36:1602–5.
[11] Douglas DD, Taswell HF, Rakela J, Rabe D. Absence of hepatitis B virus DNA detected by polymerase chain reaction in blood donors who are hepatitis B surface antigen negative and

antibody to hepatitis B core antigen positive from a United States population with a low prevalence of hepatitis B serologic markers. Transfusion 1993;33:212–6.
[12] Silva AE, McMahon BJ, Parkinson AJ, Sjogren MH, Hoofnagle JH, Di Bisceglie AM. Hepatitis B virus DNA in persons with isolated antibody to hepatitis B core antigen who subsequently received hepatitis B vaccine. Clin Infect Dis 1998;26:895–7.
[13] Chung HT, Lee STK, Lok ASF. Prevention of posttransfusion hepatitis B and C by screening for antibody to hepatitis C virus and antibody to HBcAg. Hepatology 1993;18:1045–9.
[14] Lok AS, Heathcote EJ, Hoofnagle JH. Management of hepatitis B 2000: summary of a workshop. Gastroenterology 2001;120:1828–53.
[15] Hadziyannis SJ. Hepatitis B e antigen negative chronic hepatitis B: from clinical recognition to pathogenesis and treatment. Viral Hepat Rev 1995;1:7–36.
[16] Osiowy C, Giles E. Evaluation of the INNO-LiPA HBV genotyping assay for the determination of hepatitis B virus genotype. J Clin Microbiol 2003;41:5473–7.
[17] Pawlotsky JM. Molecular diagnosis of viral hepatitis. Gastroenterology 2002;122:1554–68.
[18] Hu KQ, Vierling JM. Molecular diagnostic techniques for viral hepatitis. Gastroenterol Clin North Am 1994;23:479–98.
[19] Barlet V, Cohard M, Thelu MA, Chaix MJ, Baccard C, Zarski JP, et al. Quantitative detection of hepatitis B virus DNA in serum using chemiluminescence: comparison of radioactive solution hybridization assay. J Virol Methods 1994;49:141–51.
[20] Digene Corporation Website. Hybrid Capture Technology. Available at: http://www.digene.com/labs/labs_hybrid.html. Accessed December 18, 2005.
[21] Urdea MS, Horn T, Fultz TJ, Anderson M, Running JA, Hamren S, et al. Branched DNA amplification multimers for the sensitive, direct detection of human hepatitis viruses. Nucleic Acids Symp Ser 1991;24:197–200.
[22] Loeb KR, Jerome KR, Goddard J, Huang M, Cent A, Corey L. High-throughput quantitative analysis of hepatitis B virus DNA in serum using the TaqMan fluorogenic detection system. Hepatology 2000;32:626–9.
[23] Ho SKN, Yam W, Leung ETK, Wong L, Leung JKH, Lai K, et al. Rapid quantification of hepatitis B virus DNA by real-time PCR using fluorescent hybridization probes. J Med Micro-biol 2003;52:397–402.
[24] Higuchi R, Fockler C, Dollinger G, Watson R. Kinetic PCR analysis: real-time monitoring of DNA amplification reactions. Biotechnology (NY) 1993;11:1026–30.
[25] Sum SS, Wong DK, Yuen JC, et al. Comparison of the COBAS Taq Man HBV test with the COBAS Amplicor monitor test for measurement of hepatitis B virus DNA in serum. J Med Virol 2005;77:486–90.
[26] Heid CA, Stevens J, Livak KJ, Williams PM. Real time quantitative PCR. Genome Res 1996;6:986–94.
[27] Gibson UE, Heid CA, Williams PM. A novel method for real time quantitative RT-PCR. Genome Res 1996;6:995–1001.
[28] Saldanha J, Gerlich W, Lelie N, Dawson P, Heermann K, Heath A, WHO Collaborative Study Group. An international collaborative study to establish a World Health Organization international standard for hepatitis B virus DNA nucleic acid amplification techniques. Vox Sang 2001;80:63–71.

ELSEVIER
SAUNDERS

Infect Dis Clin N Am
20 (2006) 63–79

INFECTIOUS
DISEASE CLINICS
OF NORTH AMERICA

Assessment and Management of Chronic Hepatitis B

Marc G. Ghany, MD[a,*], Edward C. Doo, MD[b]

[a]Liver Diseases Section, National Institute of Diabetes and Digestive and Kidney Diseases, National Institutes of Health, Building 10, Room 9B-06, 10 Center Drive, MSC 1800, Bethesda, MD 29892-1800, USA

[b]Liver Disease Research Branch, National Institute of Diabetes and Digestive and Kidney Diseases, National Institutes of Health, 6707 Democracy Boulevard, MSC 5450, Bethesda, MD 20892-5450, USA

Infection with the hepatitis B virus (HBV) is a significant global public health problem. Over one third of the world population has been exposed to the virus, and an estimated 400 million people are chronically infected [1,2]. Up to 40% of chronically infected individuals will be at risk for cirrhosis, decompensated liver disease, and hepatocellular carcinoma (HCC), and each year, an estimated 500,000 deaths occur from these complications. Advances in molecular biology techniques have led to a better understanding of the natural history and pathogenesis of HBV-related liver disease, resulting in the development of potent antiviral agents. Some of these agents can be used safely as maintenance therapy for patients who fail to clear the virus following standard durations of treatment. Overall, the advent of newer therapies has provided a wider range of therapeutic options for chronic hepatitis B (CHB) infection. This article focuses on the natural history of CHB-related liver disease, assessment and selection of patients for therapy, and new therapeutic options. It is meant to provide a succinct update on the management of CHB based on recent advancements in knowledge of the disease.

A version of this article originally appeared in the 33:3 issue of Gastroenterology Clinics of North America.

* Corresponding author.
E-mail address: marcg@bldg10.niddk.nih.gov (M.G. Ghany).

0891-5520/06/$ - see front matter
doi:10.1016/j.idc.2006.01.009 *id.theclinics.com*

Natural history

The natural history of HBV infection is variable and influenced by a complex interplay between the host immune response and the replication fitness of the virus. Other factors impacting on the course of HBV infection include age at time of exposure, integrity of the immune system, alcohol consumption, obesity, and concurrent viral infections such as hepatitis C virus (HCV), hepatitis D virus (HDV), and HIV. In addition, viral load, viral variants, and perhaps HBV genotype may affect the clinical course. Ultimately, the outcome of HBV infection is determined by the robustness of the immune response as highlighted by the different clinical courses of perinatally and adult-acquired infection. Exposure at birth or at a young age when the immune system is thought to be immature represents the highest risk for developing CHB, where 90–95% of exposed infants develop chronic infection. In stark contrast, 90–95% of adult cases of HBV infection resolve spontaneously.

The natural history of HBV can be divided into 3 phases, an immune tolerant phase, an immune active phase, and an inactive phase. The immune tolerant phase is generally absent in adult acquired infection. The immune tolerant phase is characterized by a lack of symptoms, no or minimal elevation in serum aminotransferase levels and mild inflammation on liver biopsy. However, HBV DNA levels can be quite high and hepatitis B e antigen (HBeAg), a surrogate marker of viral replication is found in serum [3]. Immune tolerance is believed to be due to the inability of the host immune system to fully recognize viral antigens and may persist for 10 to 30 years [3] (Fig. 1A). During this period there is a low rate of spontaneous viral clearance.

The immune active phase is characterized by fluctuating HBV DNA levels, high serum aminotransferase levels, and hepatic necroinflammation. This phase is thought to be the result of incomplete attempts by the host immune response to eradicate virally infected hepatocytes [4] (Fig. 1B). Clinical manifestations of chronic liver disease may appear during repeated bouts of immune-mediated aminotransferase flares and may accelerate the progression of hepatic fibrosis to cirrhosis [5–7]. During these flares, a small number of patients (10–15%) may lose HBeAg spontaneously, followed by the development of antibody to HBeAg (anti-HBe), a so called HBeAg seroconversion heralding a period of quiescence in liver disease and the inactive phase [5–7]. This phase is associated with normal aminotransferase levels and less hepatic inflammation [6].

Attainment of the inactive phase has also been referred to as the transition from a high to low viral replicative status due to the marked drop in HBV DNA levels. Hepatitis B surface antigen (HBsAg), however, remains detectable in serum. The inactive phase may last for many years, and in the absence of cirrhosis, there is diminished risk for disease progression or hepatocellular carcinoma [8,9]. Thus the loss of HBeAg is an important clinical event associated with a period of disease inactivity and improved prognosis, and it

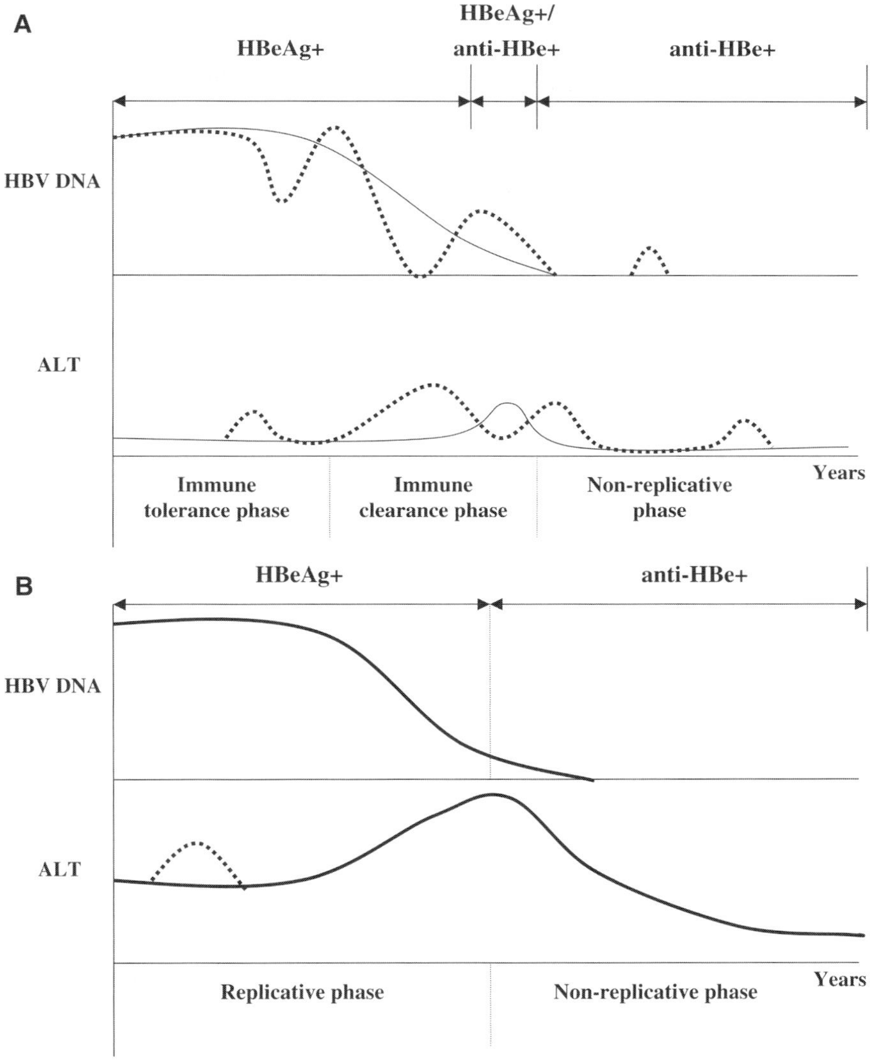

Fig. 1. Natural history of chronic HBV infection. (*dashed lines*) Represent typical fluctuations that occur with HBV infection. (*straight lines*) Represent average trends for both HBV DNA and ALT. (*A*) Course of perinatally acquired HBV infection. (*B*) Course of adult-acquired HBV infection.

often is used as an endpoint of therapy [10]. During the inactive phase, 1% to 2% of individuals per year will clear HBsAg, but as many as 30% of people may relapse back to the immunoactive phase.

Approximately 5% to 10% of individuals who lose HBeAg will continue to have detectable HBV DNA, elevated aminotransferase levels, and active inflammation on liver biopsy. These cases are defined as the HBeAg-negative or atypical form of CHB and remain in the immunoactive phase [11].

Based on this knowledge, the natural history of HBV infection can be defined by three clinical, serologic, and virologic patterns:

1. HBeAg-positive or classic CHB. This is the most common pattern and is defined by the presence of HBeAg and elevated HBV DNA in serum. The prognosis is variable and is in part dependent upon whether the infection is in the immunoactive phase (associated with elevated aminotransaminase levels and chronic hepatitis on liver biopsy) or the immunotolerant phase (associated with normal aminotransaminase levels and minimal to absent inflammation on liver biopsy).
2. HBeAg-negative or atypical CHB. This form of the infection is characterized by the absence of HBeAg but with detectable HBV DNA in serum and elevated aminotransferase levels. Features of chronic hepatitis are seen on liver biopsy, and the disease is generally active as defined by abnormal serum aminotransferase levels and liver histology [12,13]. Molecular analysis of HBV has identified the cause of this clinical presentation. Mutations in the HBV precore and core gene lead to an abrogation or reduction of HBeAg synthesis [12,13]. The clinical course can be quite severe, with more frequent episodes of acute aminotransferase flares that may lead to a greater number of liver-related complications [14]. Patients presenting with this pattern of disease should have other forms of chronic hepatitis excluded, such as hepatitis C and D infections and autoimmune and drug-induced liver disease.
3. The inactive carrier state. This is typified by the presence of anti-HBe in serum, normal alanine aminotransferase (ALT) levels, undetectable HBV DNA by hybridization assays, and minimal changes on liver biopsy. Viral replication is low in these individuals. Patients in this phase of the disease usually have a favorable prognosis and are at low risk for liver disease progression [8,15]. Occasionally, spontaneous reactivation may occur.

Assessment and monitoring

The primary goals of assessment are to determine the level of disease (active or inactive) and to stage the disease as mild, moderate, or severe. The initial evaluation of the patient should include a complete history and physical examination with particular attention directed toward eliciting signs, symptoms, and risk factors for chronic liver disease. A family history of liver disease should be sought and a detailed alcohol history obtained. Routine blood tests should include standard biochemical and hematological profiles and specific viral serologic assays for HBsAg, HBeAg, antibody to hepatitis B core antigen (anti-HBc), anti-HBe, antibody to hepatitis B surface antigen (anti-HBs), and quantitation of HBV DNA [16,17]. Which HBV DNA assay to use in clinical practice is an unresolved issue. Quantitative assays vary significantly in their sensitivity, with the lower limit of detection varying by as much as 10^3 log copies per mL. Testing for hepatitis A, C, and D and HIV should be performed routinely, as most of these viruses share similar routes of transmission as HBV, and coinfection with another virus may modify the course of HBV. Other causes of chronic liver disease should also be excluded. A baseline ultrasound examination is recommended to exclude abnormal masses or anatomical variants. A liver biopsy provides information on the grade (severity of inflammation) and the stage (severity of fibrosis) of the disease. A liver biopsy, however, can confirm the diagnosis, provide prognostic information for the patient, and assist in determining the need for therapy. Although the information gained from liver biopsy is helpful in clinical decision making, it is not an absolute requirement before treatment and should be individualized in each patient. Patients should be informed of other factors that might exacerbate progression of underlying liver disease, notably alcohol consumption, use of hepatotoxic medications, and immunosuppressants. Counseling on reducing the risk of transmission should be undertaken, especially for teenagers, young adults, and injection drug users, populations among whom the risk of sexual and parenteral transmission is high. Close family, household, and sexual contacts should be vaccinated against HBV. Individuals who do not have immunity against hepatitis A virus (HAV) should be offered hepatitis A vaccination. If bridging fibrosis or cirrhosis is found on liver biopsy, or if there is clinical evidence of advanced liver disease, a screening esophagogastroduodenoscopy is advisable to assess for portal venous hypertension via the presence of esophageal varices. Attention should be given to initiating a screening program for HCC in patients with established cirrhosis and particularly in males, older individuals, and those with a strong family history of liver cancer.

Selection of patients for treatment

There is no consensus on how to treat chronic HBV; however, several treatment guidelines have been published [16–19]. Minor differences exist in the recommendations. Identifying patients who require treatment may appear to be a straightforward task, but it is usually quite complicated in practice. There are many factors to consider in the decision-making process, including the age of the patient, stage of disease, pattern of liver disease, the patient's willingness to be treated, coinfection with other hepatotrophic viruses (HCV, HDV) and HIV, presence of other comorbid conditions and adverse effects of treatment. CHB often has a fluctuating course; therefore, after an initial assessment patients should be monitored with liver chemistries for a period of at least 6 months to assess the pattern of disease before initiating therapy (Fig. 2). Patients with inactive CHB are not

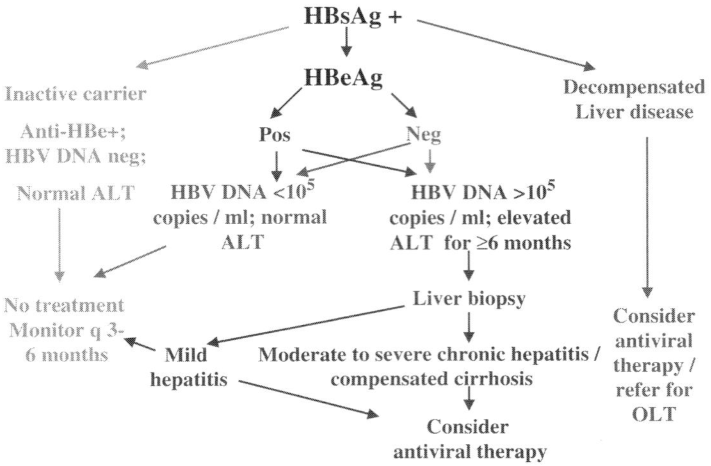

Fig. 2. Algorithm for selection of patients for therapy.

candidates for therapy. Those with mild disease as evidenced by a fibrosis score of 2 or less on the Ishak and Metavir scales or 1 on the Knodell scale and serum ALT levels persistently less than twice the upper limit of normal can defer therapy safely until more effective treatments or agents with better long-term resistance profiles become available. These patients should continue to be monitored by biochemical and serologic tests every 3 to 6 months for any evidence of acceleration of the disease. Patients with ALT elevations greater than twice the upper limit of normal, HBV DNA levels greater than 10^5 copies per mL, or with evidence of moderate-to-severe chronic hepatitis on liver biopsy are candidates for therapy. HBeAg status should be determined, as therapeutic options differ between HBeAg-positive and -negative patients. Patients with decompensated liver disease are managed best at a liver transplant center by an experienced hepatologist.

Role of hepatitis B virus genotypes

Traditionally, HBV isolates have been distinguished by serotyping based on three antigenic determinants of the HBsAg. Common to all isolates is the ‘a’ epitope and two pairs that are mutually exclusive to each other, (d or y) and (r or w), thus giving rise to four major serotypes: adr, adw, ayr, and ayw. With the advent of genetic sequencing, HBV was classified into seven genotypes (A to G) based on a nucleotide divergence in the entire genome of at least 8% [20–22]. Genotypes also can be identified by analysis of the small envelope gene of HBsAg (s-gene), where the inter-genotype divergence is of the order of 4%.

The seven genotypes have a characteristic geographical distribution, but most have a worldwide prevalence because of human migration. Of the seven genotypes, types A through D are the most common worldwide. Genotype A is found predominantly in North America, northwest Europe, and central Africa; genotypes B and C prevail in China, Japan, and Southeast Asia. Genotype D is found primarily in the Mediterranean, Middle East, and Indian subcontinent (Table 1). A recent study reported that the predominant United States genotypes were types A and C, suggesting a change in the prevalence of genotypes in the United States population. However, over 50% of patients in the study were of Asian ethnicity. Additionally, genotype A was more common in American-born patients, whereas genotype C was more common among Asian-born patients. This suggests that the increased prevalence of HBV genotype C in the United States population was most likely caused by immigration from endemic regions of the world [23].

With HCV, genotyping has been found to have an important role in managing infection. It is one of the strongest predictors of response to therapy and influences the therapeutic duration. There have been several recent studies attempting to correlate HBV genotypes with clinical parameters such as the rate of HBeAg seroconversion, development of clinically important mutations, severity of liver disease, and response to treatment.

Several studies have suggested that genotype may correlate with disease activity. When compared with genotype B, genotype C was associated with higher ALT levels and a higher prevalence of cirrhosis [24]. HBV genotype B was shown to be associated with an earlier time to HBeAg seroconversion, which may help to explain the lower disease activity reported in Asian patients [24–26], and with a higher rate of hepatocellular carcinoma in younger individuals [27]. A recent study from India found that patients with genotype D have more severe disease and a higher rate of HCC compared

Table 1
Geographical distribution and clinical relevance of hepatitis B virus genotypes

HBV genotype	Geographical distribution	Clinical relevance
A	North America, North western Europe, Central Africa	• Better response to peginterferon
B	China, Indonesia, Vietnam, Taiwan	• Lower disease activity • Associated with HCC in noncirrhotic individuals • Improved response to interferon and lamivudine
C	East Asia, Korea, China, Taiwan, Japan, Polynesia, Vietnam	• Associated with more severe liver disease
D	Mediterranean, Middle East, India	• Associated with precore mutation and HBeAg status
E	Nigeria, West Africa	Unknown
F	Alaska, Polynesia	Unknown
G	North America, France	Unknown

with patients with genotype A [28]. Given the heterogeneity of the data, it is clear that the role of HBV genotypes in relation to clinical outcome requires further investigation.

A relationship between viral burden and HBV genotype also has been suggested. Analysis of a large cohort of patients enrolled in phase III trials of adefovir showed that in HBeAg-positive CHB patients, HBV DNA levels were significantly higher in genotypes A, B, and D compared with genotype C. In contrast, among HBeAg-negative patients, significantly higher HBV DNA levels were found in those with genotype D.

The two predominant mutations that lead to HBeAg-negative CHB appear to be associated with specific HBV genotypes [24,29]. The precore mutation and the basic core promoter mutation are found more commonly with HBV genotypes D and A, respectively.

Lastly, genotype may affect the response to antiviral treatment. In Asian patients infected with genotypes B or C, interferon (IFN) was shown to be less effective in genotype C compared with genotype B infections [30]. A recent study reported a higher rate of HBeAg loss in HBV genotype A patients treated with peginterferon α2B [31]. A small European trial suggested that the response to lamivudine was better in patients with serotype ayw (corresponding to genotype D) compared with serotype adw (corresponding to genotype A) [32]. Furthermore, the rate of resistance was higher in patients with serotype adw [32]. A recent analysis suggested that genotype B was associated with a higher sustained loss of HBeAg in lamivudine-treated patients [33]. No association between genotype and response to treatment, however, was found in a larger cohort of adefovir-treated patients [34].

Much of the current data regarding the clinical implications of HBV genotypes should be viewed with some prudence. Many of the studies were small and cross-sectional, comparing two of the major genotypes with each other, either B with C or A with D, and may have been susceptible to referral bias. These issues serve to limit the generalizability of their respective findings and highlight the need for further studies to help define the clinical implications of HBV genotypes. At present, the data are insufficient to merit genotype testing as part of the evaluation of patients with CHB.

Screening for hepatocellular carcinoma

Hepatocellular carcinoma is a significant cause of morbidity and mortality in patients with CHB. There is no effective therapy for HCC. The rationale for HCC screening is to detect small, solitary lesions that may be more amenable to surgical resection or liver transplantation [35]. The benefit of this approach has not been substantiated. The best data to support a screening program in patients with HBV come from a population-based screening and surveillance study using periodic alpha fetoprotein (αFP) testing in 1487 HBsAg-positive Alaskan natives [36]. Rates of cancer in the screened group were compared with historical controls from a national cancer registry. During a 16-year period, 100 αFP elevations were detected, and 32 cancers were diagnosed; 22 patients underwent successful resection. The comparison group was comprised of 12 historical controls diagnosed before institution of the screening program. Survival rates were improved significantly in the screened population versus historical controls at 5 years (42% versus 0%) and at 10 years (30% versus 0%) [37]. Thus in this population, screening appeared to be effective in reducing mortality from HCC.

There have been no randomized controlled trials of screening for HCC. The two most widely employed modalities for screening are αFP testing and periodic ultrasound exams of the liver [36]. There are several limitations to both options. In the case of αFP, defining a standard cut-off and optimal frequency of testing is a matter of intense debate. Sensitivity of ultrasound is poor, ranging from 35% to 84%. It is highly operator-dependent, and like αFP testing, there is no consensus on how frequently the procedure should be performed. HCC has widely variable growth rates, with a doubling time of 1 to 19 months, with a median of 6 months. Thus, most authorities recommend a screening interval of 6 months.

Among histologically proven cases of HCC, 30% do not present with serum αFP elevations, and 30% of tumors smaller than 2 cm may not be detected by ultrasound. Thus, in clinical practice, both tests are used, adding to the cost of screening. Specific guidelines for screening are difficult to formulate in part because of the expense of current screening modalities, the absence of a test with suitable sensitivity and specificity, and the lack of effective therapy. Two recent conferences held on the management of CHB recommended that αFP and/or ultrasound should be performed every 6 months in patients with cirrhosis, patients older than 40 years, and those with a family history of HCC [16,17].

Treatment goals

The objectives of therapy can be viewed in terms of short- and long-term goals. Short-term objectives are to reduce viral burden, improve serum aminotransferase levels, and reduce hepatic necroinflammation. Improvement of these parameters would be expected to slow the progression of fibrosis. Long-term goals of therapy are to prevent progression to cirrhosis and HCC and ultimately improve survival. Once a decision is made to treat, the dilemmas facing the clinician are choosing which drug to use, deciding upon the optimal duration of treatment, and how to assess response to treatment. There are five approved therapies for CHB: IFN-α, peginterferon, lamivudine, adefovir dipivoxil, and entecavir. Any of these agents can be used as first-line therapy, and each is discussed in detail in separate articles within this issue. When recommending treatment, the benefits and adverse effects of each drug should be discussed, as well as the situations where one agent is favored over another. The advantages of IFN-α include a finite period of administration, lack of drug resistance and, if attained, a durable response. Patients opting for nucleoside therapy should be informed of the potential need for long-term treatment and the development of drug resistance.

Traditionally, the endpoint of therapy was loss of HBeAg and gain of anti-HBe, because seroconversion was associated with a favorable long-term prognosis after successful IFN-α treatment. This endpoint may not be suitable to assess the efficacy of nucleoside/nucleotide analog therapy because of reported relapse rates that range from 30% to 67% 2 to 3 years after therapy cessation [38–40]. At a recent NIH workshop on the management of CHB, the need for standardized definitions of response to antiviral therapy to allow for comparison of responses among different therapies was highlighted. It was recommended that response incorporate biochemical, serological, virological, and histological parameters and defined in the context of timing of treatment (ie, at initiation, during, at termination, or after termination of treatment) [16]. The remainder of this article will be devoted to a discussion on new investigative agents, highlighting those that appear to be most promising (Table 2).

Promising new hepatitis B agents

Tenofovir

Tenofovir disoproxil fumarate is the prodrug of tenofovir and is a nucleoside analog approved as an antiretroviral agent. Tenofovir has been shown to exhibit antiviral activity against HBV [41]. In patients coinfected with HIV and HBV where tenofovir was added as a component of antiretroviral therapy, HBV viral load decreased by approximately 4 log after 1 year of therapy [42]. Tenofovir appears to remain effective against the lamivudine HBV polymerase mutant [43,44]. Additionally, in patients with HIV/HBV coinfection who were HBeAg negative, short-term treatment with tenofovir led to a reduction of HBV viral titers [45]. Thus, tenofovir may be a potential adjunctive therapeutic agent against CHB infection in patients coinfected with HIV. Additional studies are needed to evaluate the potential of tenofovir as monotherapy for CHB infection. Renal toxicity has been reported with tenofovir.

Emtricitabine

Emtricitabine (FTC, 2′3′-dideoxy-5′fluoro-3′-thiacytidine) is a nucleoside analog that is structurally similar to lamivudine. An initial in vitro study demonstrated inhibition of HBV replication by emtricitabine [47]. Significant reductions in woodchuck hepatitis virus (WHV) titers with emtricitabine were observed in chronically infected woodchucks [48]. The antiviral effect also was observed in people in a phase I clinical trial [49].

Table 2
New compounds in development for treatment of chronic hepatitis B infection

Generic name	Molecular structure	Phase of development	Activity against lamivudine resistant strains	Resistance reported
Clevudine	2′-fluoro-5-methyl-L-arabinofuranosyl uracil nucleoside analogue	Phase II	No	Yes
Emtricitabine	2′3′dideoxy-5′fluoro-3′-thiacytidine nucleoside analogue	?Phase III	No	Yes
Lobucavir	Carbocyclic analogue of oxetanocin	Phase I., studies terminated because to toxicity in rodents	Unknown	Unknown
Tenofovir	Adenosine nucleotide analogue	Phase III	Yes	No
Amdoxovir	D-2,6-diaminopurine dioxolane	Phase I	Unclear	Unknown
Beta-L-nucleosides	Beta-L-thymidine	Phase I		Unknown
Heteroaryldihydropyrimidines	Same		Unknown	Unknown

Preliminary results from a placebo-controlled phase 3 study in treatment naïve patients has demonstrated that 48 weeks of emtricitabine (200 mg daily) reduces serum HBV DNA by a median of 3^{10} copies per mL and significantly improves liver histology [50]. The drug is structurally similar to lamiveudine and shares similar mutational sites and rate of resistance. The incidence of resistance is 9–6% at week 96 [51]. Given these findings it is unlikely this drug will play a major role in the management of chronic HBV.

Clevudine

Clevudine (L-FMAU, 2′-fluoro-5-methyl-β-L-arabinofuranosyl uracil) is a pyrimidine nucleoside analog that has been demonstrated to have antiviral effects in short-term studies with woodchucks chronically infected with WHV [52]. In chronically infected woodchucks, however, prolonged therapy with L-FMAU resulted in viral rebound cause by the development of resistant WHV polymerase mutants [53]. In a small human pilot study evaluating four doses of clevudine (10 mg, 50 mg, 100 mg, and 200 mg) for 4 weeks, the mean reduction in HBV DNA level was −2.5 to −3.0 log for all doses tested. The reduction in HBV DNA was sustained up to 24 weeks after cessation of treatment and was highest in the 100 mg dose group (−2.7 logs). Of treated patients, 19% had loss of HBeAg, and few adverse effects were reported. No mitochondrial toxicity was observed. A phase III trial of clevudine 3 mg orally daily for 24 weeks followed by 24 weeks of followup showed 59% of undetectable virus and 68% with ALT normalization. No viral breakthrough was noted during therapy. Final results are pending.

Beta-L-nucleosides

Beta-L-nucleosides are potential therapeutic antiviral agents against HBV being evaluated in duck hepatitis virus and WHV models. There are three of these analogs under investigation: LdC (beta-L-2′-deoxycytidine; valtorcitabine), LdT (beta-L-thymidine, telbivudine), and LdA (beta-L-2′-deoxyadenosine). All have demonstrated specificity for the HBV polymerase, and LdT is being evaluated in clinical trials [54].

Telbivudine

Telbivudine (Ldt) is a beta-L-nucleoside that is currently in Phase III trials. Initial studies demonstrated the potent activity of LdT against HBV in in vitro studies. Results of a Phase II trial with LdT in varying doses as monotherapy and in combination with lamivudine demonstrated significantly more reduction in HBV DNA in treatment arms that contained LdT than with lamivudine monotherapy. The rate of HBV genotypic resistance to LdT is not insignificant and was reported to be 4.5% after one year and rose to 18.2% after 96 weeks of therapy.

Antiviral agents requiring further investigation

Lobucavir

Lobucavir is a carbocyclic analog of oxetanocin shown to be an effective antiviral agent against HBV [46]. Further studies were terminated when hepatic and foregut tumors emerged during long-term rodent carcinogenesis studies.

Amdoxovir

Amdoxovir (DAPD, β-D-2,6-diaminopurine dioxolane) is a prodrug of 1-β-D-dioxolane (DXG), which has antiretroviral activity against HIV-1 [55]. In vitro studies of amdoxovir sensitivity among lamivudine-resistant HBV polymerase mutant strains are inconsistent, and additional studies will be needed to clarify DAPD's utility in this setting [56]. Amdoxovir is currently being evaluated in phase I/II studies of HIV-positive patients.

Pradefovir

Pradefovir mesylate (PDV) is a cyclodiester prodrug of adefovir that is biotransformed in heptocytes by the cytochrome P450 3A4 into the active compound. The premise of this approach is to use higher doses that concentrate into infected hepatocytes while sparing renal tubule toxicity. Interim results at 24 weeks of therapy of a Phase II study in patients with lamivudine resistant HBV, pradefovir at a dose of 30 mg appeared to be equivalent to standard adefovir. The caveat is that the number of patients analyzed was small and the results will need to be reassessed once the study matures.

Heteroaryldihydropyrimidines

Heteroaryldihydropyrimidines (HAPs) are compounds that effectively inhibit HBV replication at the level of viral capsid assembly. Critical molecular events in the life cycle of HBV occur within the milieu of the assembled capsid, including synthesis of the genome [57]. Initial in vitro studies have demonstrated that HAPs disrupt the formation of viral capsids by enhancing proteasome-mediated degradation of capsid monomers [58]. Future studies with these compounds are awaited, as they may represent a novel approach to HBV treatment.

Other novel approaches

Several novel approaches are being developed for treating hepatitis B. Several immunotherapeutic strategies have been tried in an attempt to modulate the immune response either alone or in combination with antiviral agents [59]. HBsAg vaccination, in combination with lamivudine and a lipopeptide-based T-cell vaccine designed to induce a core-specific cytotoxic T-lymphocyte (CTL) response, has been used in clinical trials, albeit without much success. Another novel approach to inhibit viral replication has been through the development of antisense oligonucleotides and hammerhead ribosomes. Both of these agents form hybridization duplexes with specific target viral mRNA sequences, ultimately leading to viral RNA degradation either through activation of host RNaseH or intrinsic catalytic activity. Several technical issues hinder practical use of this technology in the treatment of HBV infection, such as transport into target cells, absence of target tissue specificity, degradation by host enzymes, and poor bioavailability. Most recently, small interfering RNAs have been shown in cell culture to reduce the level of viral transcripts and proteins and replicative forms [60]. Many technical issues will need to be addressed before these potential therapeutic modalities become feasible.

Summary

An understanding of the natural history of CHB is critical for the management of the liver disease. Three clinical patterns with different clinical outcomes are recognized: HBeAg-positive CHB, HBeAg-negative CHB, and inactive CHB. Patients with elevated aminotransferase levels and HBV DNA greater than 10^5 viral copies per mL in serum and with features of chronic hepatitis on liver biopsy are candidates for therapy regardless of HBeAg status. Multiple host and viral factors and safety profiles of current therapies need to be considered carefully before recommending therapy. There appears to be no role for HBV genotyping in the management of patients. Three antiviral agents are approved for use against CHB infection: IFN-α, lamivudine, and adefovir. Efficacy is moderate at best and is limited by the poor tolerability of IFN and the development of resistance, coupled with concerns regarding the long-term safety with nucleoside analogs. Several new nucleoside and nucleotide analogs and novel agents are at various stages of development as potential therapies for CHB. The ideal compound would be one that is active against all replicative intermediates of the virus and has a low toxicity profile. Despite current shortcomings, the future of therapy for HBV is promising, as newer therapeutic options are being developed based on an understanding of the HBV life cycle.

References

[1] World Health Organization Fact Sheet/204. Hepatitis B. Geneva: World Health Organization; 2000.

[2] Lee WM. Hepatitis B virus infection. N Engl J Med 1997;337(24):1733–45.

[3] Lok AS, Lai CL. A longitudinal follow-up of asymptomatic hepatitis B surface antigen-positive Chinese children. Hepatology 1988;8(5):1130–3.

[4] Guidotti LG, Rochford R, Chung J, Shapiro M, Purcell R, Chisari FV. Viral clearance without destruction of infected cells during acute HBV infection. Science 1999;284(5415): 825–9.

[5] Hoofnagle JH, Dusheiko GM, Seeff LB, Jones EA, Waggoner JG, Bales ZB. Seroconversion from hepatitis B e antigen to antibody in chronic type B hepatitis. Ann Intern Med 1981; 94(6):744–8.

[6] Di Bisceglie AM, Waggoner JG, Hoofnagle JH. Hepatitis B virus deoxyribonucleic acid in liver of chronic carriers. Correlation with serum markers and changes associated with loss of hepatitis B e antigen after antiviral therapy. Gastroenterology 1987;93(6):1236–41.

[7] Realdi G, Alberti A, Rugge M, et al. Seroconversion from hepatitis B e antigen to anti-HBe in chronic hepatitis B virus infection. Gastroenterology 1980;79(2):195–9.

[8] de Franchis R, Meucci G, Vecchi M, Tatarella M, Colombo M, Del Ninno E, et al. The natural history of asymptomatic hepatitis B surface antigen carriers. Ann Intern Med 1993; 118(3):191–4.

[9] de Jongh FE, Janssen HL, de Man RA, Hop WC, Schalm SW, van Blankenstein M. Survival and prognostic indicators in hepatitis B surface antigen-positive cirrhosis of the liver. Gastroenterology 1992;103(5):1630–5.

[10] Hoofnagle JH, Shafritz DA, Popper H. Chronic type B hepatitis and the healthy HBsAg carrier state. Hepatology 1987;7(4):758–63.

[11] Hadziyannis SJ, Vassilopoulos D. Hepatitis B e antigen-negative chronic hepatitis B. Hepatology 2001;34:617–24.

[12] Carman WF, Jacyna MR, Hadziyannis S, Karayiannis P, McGarvey MJ, Makris A, et al. Mutation preventing formation of hepatitis B e antigen in patients with chronic hepatitis B infection. Lancet 1989;2(8663):588–91.

[13] Brunetto MR, Stemler M, Bonino F, Schodel F, Oliveri F, Rizzetto M, et al. A new hepatitis B virus strain in patients with severe anti-HBe-positive chronic hepatitis B. J Hepatol 1990; 10(2):258–61.

[14] Hadziyannis S. Hepatitis B e antigen-negative chronic hepatitis B: from clinical recognition to pathogenesis and treatment. Viral Hepatitis Review 1995;1:7–36.

[15] Hsu YS, Chien RN, Yeh CT, Sheen IS, Chiou HY, Chu CM, et al. Long-term outcome after spontaneous HBeAg seroconversion in patients with chronic hepatitis B. Hepatology 2002; 35(6):1522–7.

[16] Lok AS, Heathcote EJ, Hoofnagle JH. Management of hepatitis B: 2000—summary of a workshop. Gastroenterology 2001;120(7):1828–53.

[17] EASL International Consensus Conference on Hepatitis B. 13–14 September, 2002: Geneva, Switzerland. Consensus statement (short version). J Hepatol 2003;38(4):533–40.

[18] Lok AS, McMahon BJ. Practice Guidelines Committee, American Association for the Study of Liver Diseases. Chronic hepatitis B. Hepatology 2001;34(6):1225–41.

[19] Keeffe EB, Dieterich DT, Han SH, et al. A treatment algorithm for the management of chronic hepatitis B virus infection in the United States. Clin Gastroenterol Hepatol 2004; 2(2):87–106.

[20] Okamoto H, Tsuda F, Sakugawa H, Sastrosoenignjo RI, Imai M, Miyakana Y, et al. Typing hepatitis B virus by homology in nucleotide sequence: comparison of surface antigen subtypes. J Gen Virol 1988;69:2575–83.

[21] Norder H, Courouce AM, Magnius LO. Complete genomes, phylogenetic relatedness, and structural proteins of six strains of the hepatitis B virus, four of which represent two new genotypes. Virology 1994;198(2):489–503.

[22] Stuyver L, De Gendt S, Van Geyt C, Zoulim F, Fried M, Schinazi RF, et al. A new genotype of hepatitis B virus: complete genome and phylogenetic relatedness. J Gen Virol 2000; 81(Pt 1):67–74.

[23] Chu CJ, Keeffe EB, Han SH, Perello RP, Min AD, Soldevila-Pico C, et al. Hepatitis B virus genotypes in the United States: results of a nationwide study. Gastroenterology 2003;125(2): 444–51.

[24] Lindh M, Hannoun C, Dhillon AP, Norkrans G, Horal P. Core promoter mutations and genotypes in relation to viral replication and liver damage in East Asian hepatitis B virus carriers. J Infect Dis 1999;179(4):775–82.
[25] Chu CJ, Hussain M, Lok AS. Hepatitis B virus genotype B is associated with earlier HBeAg seroconversion compared with hepatitis B virus genotype C. Gastroenterology 2002;122(7): 1756–62.
[26] Orito E, Mizokami M, Sakugawa H, Michitaka K, Ishikana K, Iehida T, et al. Acase-control study for clinical and molecular biological differences between hepatitis B viruses of genotypes B and C. Japan HBV Genotype Research Group. Hepatology 2001;33(1):218–23.
[27] Kao JH, Chen PJ, Lai MY, Chen DS. Hepatitis B genotypes correlate with clinical outcomes in patients with chronic hepatitis B. Gastroenterology 2000;118(3):554–9.
[28] Thakur V, Guptan RC, Kazim SN, Malhotra V, Sarin SK. Profile, spectrum and significance of HBV genotypes in chronic liver disease patients in the Indian subcontinent. J Gastroenterol Hepatol 2002;17(2):165–70.
[29] Rodriguez-Frias F, Buti M, Jardi R, Cotrina M, Viladomina L, Esteban R, et al. Hepatitis B virus infection: precore mutants and its relation to viral genotypes and core mutations. Hepatology 1995;22(6):1641–7.
[30] Kao JH, Wu NH, Chen PJ, Lai MY, Chen DS. Hepatitis B genotypes and the response to interferon therapy. J Hepatol 2000;33(6):998–1002.
[31] Janssen HL, van Zonneveld M, Senturk H, et al. Pegylated interferon alfa-2b alone or in combination with lamivudine for HBeAg-positive chronic hepatitis B: a randomised trail. Lancet 2005;365(9454):123–9.
[32] Zollner B, Petersen J, Schroter M, Laufs R, Schoder V, Feucht HH. 20-fold increase in risk of lamivudine resistance in hepatitis B virus subtype adw. Lancet 2001;357(9260):934–5.
[33] Chien RN, Yeh CT, Tsai SL, Chu CM, Liaw YF. Determinants for sustained HBeAg response to lamivudine therapy. Hepatology 2003;38(5):1267–73.
[34] Westland C, Delaney WT, Yang H, Chen SS, Marcellin P, Hadziyannis S, et al. Hepatitis B virus genotypes and virologic response in 694 patients in phase III studies of adefovir dipivoxil1. Gastroenterology 2003;125(1):107–16.
[35] Mazzaferro V, Regalia E, Doci R, Andreola S, Palvirenti A, Bozzetti F, et al. Liver transplantation for the treatment of small hepatocellular carcinomas in patients with cirrhosis. N Engl J Med 1996;334(11):693–9.
[36] McMahon BJ, Bulkow L, Harpster A, Snowball M, Lanier A, Sacco F, et al. Screening for hepatocellular carcinoma in Alaska natives infected with chronic hepatitis B: a 16-year population-based study. Hepatology 2000;32:842–6.
[37] McMahon BJ, London T. Workshop on screening for hepatocellular carcinoma. J Natl Cancer Inst 1991;83(13):916–9.
[38] van Nunen AB, Hansen BE, Suh DJ, Lohr HF, Chemello L, Fontaine H, et al. Durability of HBeAg seroconversion following antiviral therapy for chronic hepatitis B: relation to type of therapy and pretreatment serum hepatitis B virus DNA and alanine aminotransferase. Gut 2003;52(3):420–4.
[39] Song BC, Suh DJ, Lee HC, Chung YH, Lee YS. Hepatitis B e antigen seroconversion after lamivudine therapy is not durable in patients with chronic hepatitis B in Korea. Hepatology 2000;32:803–6.
[40] Dienstag JL, Cianciara J, Karayalcin S, Kowdley KV, Willems B, Plisek S, et al. Durability of serologic response after lamivudine treatment of chronic hepatitis B. Hepatology 2003; 37(4):748–55.
[41] Ying C, De Clercq E, Neyts J. Lamivudine, adefovir and tenofovir exhibit long-lasting anti-hepatitis B virus activity in cell culture. J Viral Hepat 2000;7(1):79–83.
[42] Nelson M, Portsmouth S, Stebbing J, Atkins M, Burr A, Matthews G, et al. An open-label study of tenofovir in HIV-1 and Hepatitis B virus coinfected individuals. AIDS 2003;17(1): F7–10.

[43] Ying C, De Clercq E, Nicholson W, Furman P, Neyts J. Inhibition of the replication of the DNA polymerase M550V mutation variant of human hepatitis B virus by adefovir, tenofovir, L-FMAU, DAPD, penciclovir and lobucavir. J Viral Hepat 2000;7(2):161–5.
[44] Benhamou Y, Tubiana R, Thibault V. Tenofovir disoproxil fumarate in patients with HIV and lamivudine-resistant hepatitis B virus. N Engl J Med 2003;348(2):177–8.
[45] Bruno R, Sacchi P, Zocchetti C, Ciappina V, Puoti M, Filice G. Rapid hepatitis B virus-DNA decay in co-infected HIV-hepatitis B virus e-minus patients with YMDD mutations after 4 weeks of tenofovir therapy. AIDS 2003;17(5):783–4.
[46] Bloomer J, Chen R, Sherman M, Ingraham P, De Hertogh D. A preliminary study of lobucavir for chronic hepatitis B. Hepatology 1997;26:A1199.
[47] Doong SL, Tsai CH, Schinazi RF, Liotta DC, Cheng YC. Inhibition of the replication of hepatitis B virus in vitro by 2′,3′-dideoxy-3′-thiacytidine and related analogues. Proc Natl Acad Sci U S A 1991;88(19):8495–9.
[48] Korba BE, Schinazi RF, Cote P, Tennant BC, Gerin JL. Effect of oral administration of emtricitabine on woodchuck hepatitis virus replication in chronically infected woodchucks. Antimicrob Agents Chemother 2000;44(6):1757–60.
[49] Gish RG, Leung NW, Wright TL, Trinh H, Lang N, Kessler HA, et al. Dose range study of pharmacokinetics, safety, and preliminary antiviral activity of emtricitabine in adults with hepatitis B virus infection. Antimicrob Agents Chemother 2002;46(6):1734–40.
[50] Shiffman ML, et al. AASLD 2004 [abstract 22].
[51] Gish. AASLD 2002 [abstract 838].
[52] Chu CK, Boudinot FD, Peek SF, Hong JH, Choi Y, Korba BE, et al. Preclinical investigation of L-FMAU as an antihepatitis B virus agent. Antivir Ther 1998;3(Suppl 3):113–21.
[53] Zhu Y, Yamamoto T, Cullen J, Saputelli J, Aldrich CE, Miller DS, et al. Kinetics of hepadnavirus loss from the liver during inhibition of viral DNA synthesis. J Virol 2001;75(1): 311–22.
[54] Mewshaw JP, Myrick FT, Wakefield DA, Hooper BJ, Harris JL, McCrudy B, et al. Dioxolane guanosine, the active form of the prodrug diaminopurine dioxolane, is a potent inhibitor of drug-resistant HIV-1 isolates from patients for whom standard nucleoside therapy fails. J Acquir Immune Defic Syndr 2002;29(1):11–20.
[55] Seigneres B, Pichoud C, Martin P, Furman P, Trepo C, Zoulim F. Inhibitory activity of dioxolane purine analogs on wild-type and lamivudine-resistant mutants of hepadnaviruses. Hepatology 2002;36(3):710–22.
[56] Standring DN, Bridges EG, Placidi L, Faraj A, Loi AG, Pierra C, et al. Antiviral beta-L-nucleosides specific for hepatitis B virus infection. Antivir Chem Chemother 2001;12(Suppl 1): 119–29.
[57] Doo E, Liang TJ. Molecular anatomy and pathophysiologic implications of drug resistance in hepatitis B virus infection. Gastroenterology 2001;120(4):1000–8.
[58] Deres K, Schroder CH, Paessens A, Goldman S, Hacker HJ, Weber O, et al. Inhibition of hepatitis B virus replication by drug-induced depletion of nucleocapsids. Science 2003; 299(5608):893–6.
[59] Michel ML, Pol S, Brechot C, Tiollais P. Immunotherapy of chronic hepatitis B by anti-HBV vaccine: from present to future. Vaccine 2001;19:2395–9.
[60] Shlomai A, Shaul Y. Inhibition of hepatitis B virus expression and replication by RNA interference. Hepatology 2003;37(4):764–70.

ELSEVIER
SAUNDERS

Infect Dis Clin N Am
20 (2006) 81–98

INFECTIOUS
DISEASE CLINICS
OF NORTH AMERICA

Molecular Virology of the Hepatitis C Virus: Implication for Novel Therapies

Jeffrey S. Glenn, MD, PhD

Division of Gastroenterology and Hepatology, Stanford University School of Medicine and Palo Alto Veterans Administration Medical Center, CCSR Building, Room 3115, 269 Campus Drive, Palo Alto, CA 94305-5187, USA

Hepatitis C virus (HCV) is a significant cause of morbidity and mortality, infecting over 150 million people worldwide [1,2]. In spite of recent progress, current therapies remain inadequate for the majority of patients [3–5]. The study of HCV molecular virology is providing an increasing number of new anti-HCV targets. These are being translated into the development of new drugs that offer the prospect of more effective antiviral therapies. This article provides a concise review and update of the major highlights in these efforts.

Overview of life cycle

HCV is a positive, single-stranded, RNA virus. Its 9.6-kb genome encodes a single ~3000 amino acid polyprotein that is proteolytically processed by a combination of cellular and viral proteinases into structural (components of the mature virus) and nonstructural (elements proposed to help replicate new virions) proteins (Fig. 1) [6–8]. Flanking this long protein-encoding sequence are conserved nontranslated regions at the 5′ and 3′ ends of the RNA genome. These contain highly structured elements that represent important cis-acting signals for initiating replication and translation of the viral genome.

The structural proteins include the core and envelope proteins. The core protein is thought to serve as a nucleocapsid protein. It also seems to interact with several host cell signaling pathways and has been implicated in steatosis. The core protein and the viral RNA genome are encapsulated in

A version of this article originally appeared in the 9:3 issue of Clinics in Liver Disease.

E-mail address: jeffrey.glenn@stanford.edu

doi:10.1016/j.idc.2006.01.001

id.theclinics.com

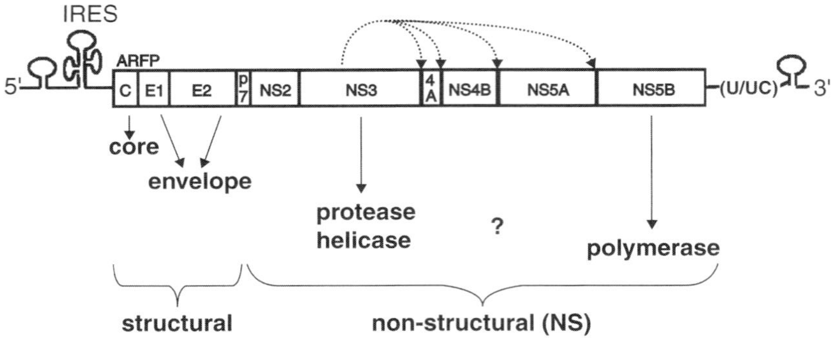

Fig. 1. Schematic of HCV genome. The 9.6-kb (+) strand RNA genome is translated beginning from an IRES into a single polyprotein (indicated by a box), 5′ and 3′ non-coding regions contain RNA elements required for genome replication. Individual proteins are liberated by a combination of host signal peptidase (N-terminal cleavages) and viral protease activity (indicated by arrows above polyprotein). Known activities of selected proteins are indicated below them.

a lipid envelope in which the two HCV envelope proteins, El and E2, are embedded. A characteristic of all viruses that, like HCV, replicate via an RNA-dependent RNA polymerase, is a relatively high rate of spontaneous mutations (presumably due to the lack of an editing function of the polymerase). The resulting genetic heterogeneity means that the virus present at any given time in an individual is best thought of as a population of related but slightly different and ever-changing genomes. This pool, or quasispecies, provides the virus with an increased ability to respond to changing selective pressures that arise from the host's immune response or the administration of antiviral drugs. The heterogeneity is particularly pronounced in certain regions of the genome, such as the hypervariable region of E2, and can pose special challenges in the areas of vaccine development and drug resistance.

Our understanding of the function of individual nonstructural proteins is better for some than others. For example, based in part on the presence of characteristic amino acid sequence motifs, enzymatic activities for NS3 and NS5B were deduced early on. Thus, NS3 has a protease activity responsible for liberating itself and the downstream nonstructural (NS) proteins from the polyprotein precursor, and NS5B encodes the catalytic activity for RNA-directed RNA polymerization. The precise roles of other NS proteins, such as NS4B and NS5A, in the HCV life cycle have been less well defined. However, they have some interesting properties, are critical for RNA replication, and are yielding attractive new targets for anti-HCV strategies.

A simplified schematic of the viral life cycle is presented in Fig. 2. Even after 15 years of intensive research since the first molecular cloning of the HCV genome, many critical details remain to be filled in. The precise mechanism of viral entry has not been defined, although several candidate

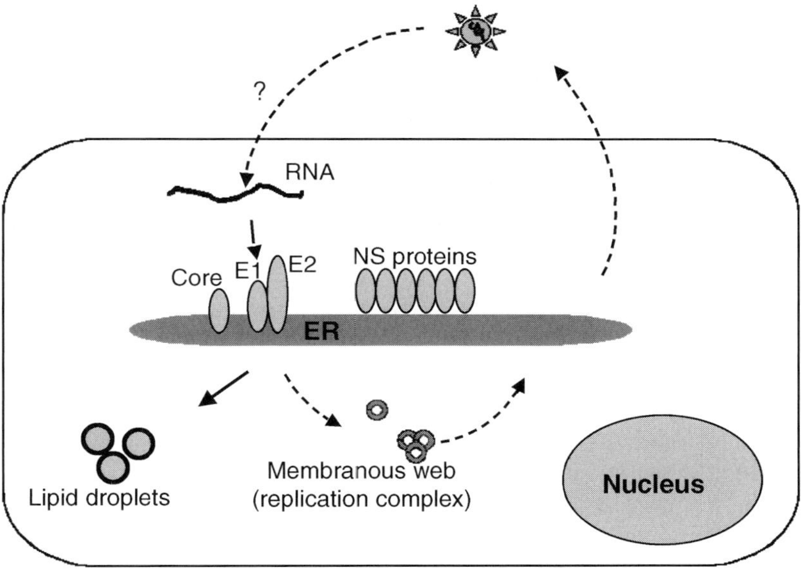

Fig. 2. Schematic of HCV life cycle. An HCV particle attaches and gains entrance to its host cell. This is thought to involve a specific receptor(s) and membrane fusion event. The use of dotted lines for various stages of the life cycle is meant to convey that many mechanistic details remain to be clarified.

receptors, or co-receptors, have been proposed [9–12]. Upon entry, uncoating of the viral genome occurs and it gains access to the host cell's translational machinery by use of an internal ribosome entry site (IRES) near the 5′ end of the genome. Initial translation and protcolytic processing occur on the endoplasmic reticulum. A novel intracellular membrane structure termed the "membranous web" is established and seems to be the platform upon which RNA replication occurs [13]. A minus strand RNA is made first that serves as template for the transcription of progeny plus strand RNA genomes, which are packaged and released in the form of new virions. The major steps in these processes occur in the host cell's cytoplasm. Several viral proteins localize to lipid droplets and, under certain circumstances, may be able to gain access to the cell's nucleus, although the significance of these events for the viral life cycle is not clear.

Molecular virology and antiviral implications

Current therapy for HCV consists of interferon (IFN) and ribavirin (RBV). These agents were already developed for other indications before HCV was first identified. In that sense they are not specific for HCV. Although IFN has anti-HCV activity by itself, the benefit of RBV is achieved only when it is used in combination with IFN. In light of their nonspecific nature, it is somewhat remarkable that impressive improvements in response rates have been achieved with these agents. This can be mainly attributed to the optimization of formulations and regimens and to the use of combination therapy. This therapy remains expensive, lengthy, and with significant side effects—all of which combine to limit its application to many patients. More importantly, current therapy is frequently ineffective.

Ultimate pharmacologic control of HCV is likely best achieved by a cocktail consisting of multiple agents against independent, virus-specific targets. Improved understanding of HCV molecular virology can play a critical role in helping to develop this more effective therapy. Such knowledge can be translated into new antiviral strategies by increasing the repertoire of potential targets that may serve as the basis for novel therapies.

One can consider three generations of anti-HCV therapy (Fig. 3). The first consists of currently approved (and nonspecific) drugs (eg, IFN and RBV), The second generation of therapy includes agents that for the first time are designed against HCV-specific targets. Several such compounds are the subject of active preclinical drug development programs. Finally, an increasing number of promising new targets are being identified at an exciting pace. These are expected to form the basis of a third generation of therapy—therapies of the future. In the following section, a survey of individual viral elements is presented, focusing on potential implications for the design of novel anti-HCV strategies.

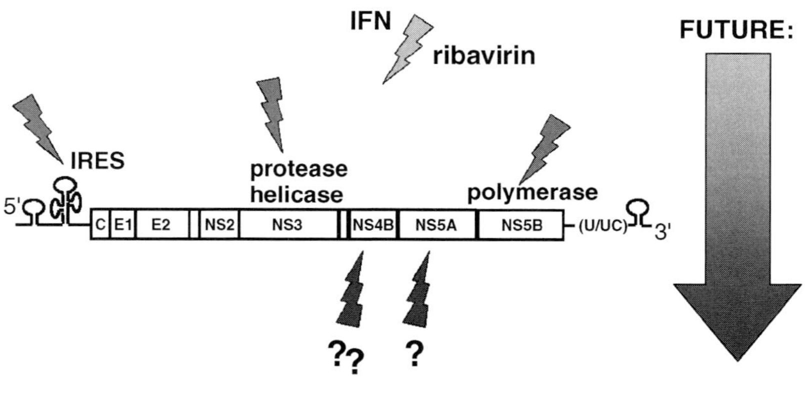

Fig. 3. Three generations of anti-HCV therapy can be defined. First generation therapies are those that are currently approved, consist of interferon and ribavirin, were available before the identification of the HCV genome, and are thus not really specific for HCV. Second generation agents are those that are specifically designed against HCV targets (such as the protease and polymerase) and are in various stages of advanced development. Third generation agents consist of the therapies of the future, and increased knowledge of HCV molecular virology is expected to expand their number. Ultimate effective pharmacologic control of HCV is likely to result from combination therapy with a cocktail of multiple drugs, each targeting an independent virus-specific function.

Core protein

The first product to be liberated from the HCV polyprotein is the core protein. The latter has been extensively studied in a variety of heterologous expression systems and has been shown to interact with a number of important host cell intracellular signaling pathways [14–18]. The precise role of these interactions in HCV pathogenesis and replication needs to be further clarified, but this raises the possibility that specific inhibition of core's interface with these signaling pathways may have important therapeutic effects.

Another core function is its presumed role in assembly. Recombinant core protein has the ability to assemble into higher-order particles [19,20], suggesting the existence of an ordered capsid structure. By analogy with HBV [21], agents capable of interfering with core particle assembly can be imagined, although much needs to be learned about natural HCV particle morphogenesis.

Many key proteins involved in intracellular signaling are localized to a specialized subdomain of host cell membranes termed lipid rafts. These lipid rafts, or detergent-resistant membranes (DRMs), are defined by their enrichment in cholesterol and resistance to solubilization with cold, nonionic detergents. Not only do lipid rafts serve as a platform for intracellular signaling, but a variety of viruses exploit lipid rafts to help mediate their assembly [22]. Recently, it was demonstrated that a subpopulation of HCV core protein in cells harboring full-length HCV replicons is biochemically associated with DRM in a manner similar to markers of classical lipid rafts [23]. This finding provides a basis for how core may accomplish its signaling and assembly functions. Moreover, the mechanism by which core protein associates with its lipid raft domain might offer a new target for antiviral intervention.

Alternate reading frame protein

All of the HCV proteins mentioned so far are translated off of one long open reading frame. It has recently been shown that at least one protein can also be translated in a second reading frame off the same HCV genomic RNA template. This later protein, termed "alternate reading frame protein" (ARFP), comes about as a result of a frameshift event in the core region of the genome [24,25]. Antibodies and evidence of cell-mediated immunity [26] against it have been found in HCV-infected patient sera. The function of the ARFP in the HCV life cycle—and validation of its requirement for productive infection—await further definition before ARFP can be considered a potential antiviral target.

E1/E2

The HCV envelope proteins El and E2 are liberated from the viral polyprotein by host signal peptidase and undergo extensive glycosylation. The two envelope proteins form a noncovalent heterodimer [27]. The membrane translocation signal sequences for El and E2 are contained within the C-terminal ends of core and El, respectively [28,29]. Upon cleavage by signal peptidase, the El and E2 C-termini undergo a reorientation in the endoplasmic reticulum (ER) membrane toward the cytosol [29].

The surface envelope proteins of viruses have frequently been used as classic elements of traditional vaccines. Effective, broad-spectrum, neutralizing antibodies against HCV using this traditional approach have been difficult to obtain. This may be related to a high rate of viral mutation of epitopes targeted by the host humoral response. Research in this area has been hampered by the lack of an efficient culture system capable of producing, and being infected with, HCV virions. The ability to make chimeric, or so-called "pseudotyped," viruses having a surface coat of HCV envelope proteins and inner replication machinery of a retrovirus [30] should help accelerate the search for neutralizing therapeutics. The latter may include drugs designed to inhibit the initial stages of viral attachment and entry. Effective vaccines of the future may also include other viral immunogens, including ones selected from conserved epitopes in the NS proteins. This may be important for stimulating optimal cellular immunity.

p7

This small (63-amino-acid) protein lies between the structural and nonstructural proteins. Similar to the viroporin M2 of influenza A virus, HCV p7 seems to function as an ion channel and is sensitive to inhibition by amantadine [31]. As such, p7 may be well suited for small molecule inhibitors, especially because its function seems to be essential for in vivo infectivity [32].

NS2

NS2 participates in the proteolytic cleavage reaction between itself and NS3 [33]. It is not required for RNA replication in model culture systems [34,35], but it may play a role in assembly. The protease reaction in which NS2 participates is a potential target for inhibition whose importance may be better appreciated with improved HCV culture systems capable of producing infectious particles. In addition, NS2 may have distinct functions when in a partially versus completely processed state. Such incompletely processed precursors are known to play important roles in other positive-strand polyprotein viruses.

NS3

NS3 is a 630-amino-acid protein that has two domains with different enzymatic activities that are thought to be essential for the HCV life cycle. The amino terminal segment has a serine protease activity, whereas the remaining two thirds have an RNA helicase activity. The protease activity is most efficient when combined with NS4A, which serves as a noncovalent cofactor and promotes the membrane association of NS3. This complex is responsible for liberating the downstream NS proteins from the initial polyprotein precursor.

The helicase activity is presumably required to help facilitate the unwinding of duplex RNA during replication of the viral genome. The crystal structures of each isolated NS3 domain and the complete molecule with and without the NS4A cofactor segment have been solved [36–39]. This has greatly facilitated the ability to perform rational drug design and optimization. These atomic structures have also revealed some potential challenges for obtaining potent inhibitors. For example, the active site of the protease is a relatively shallow cleft without prominent features that readily lend themselves to facile design of highly selective complementary chemical entities.

Several companies have NS3 protease inhibitors in advanced development. Two pharmacologically effective approaches have been taken. One is based on the finding that the products of the NS3 protease reaction are inhibitory to the enzyme. This has driven a peptidomimetric strategy whereby the inhibitor resembles a peptide within the active site of the NS3 protease. An oral-optimized inhibitor of this type was shown to decrease HCV titers by up to several logs in patients, providing successful proof-of-concept [40]. Further clinical development of this compound has been halted due to unanticipated cardiotoxicity in animal studies [41]. Although this toxicity may not be related to NS3 inhibition per se but rather to a compound-specific phenotype, it is likely that other NS3 protease inhibitors will be required to undergo cardiotoxicity screens.

A second strategy taken to develop NS3 protease inhibitors exploits the fact that this viral protease is in the class of serine proteases. Here, a so-called serine trap moiety, or "warhead," capable of covalently binding the catalytic serine, is incorporated into the final compound [42].

Although the first two NS3 protease inhibitors to enter human trials may not be those to enter clinical practice, the relatively rapid development of these compounds highlights the value that detailed structural knowledge of the target can provide. This structural information should continue to guide the development of new types of inhibitors, and it will be useful in helping us to understand the nature of potential resistance to future compounds.

The NS3 helicase function might also be considered an antiviral target [43], assuming specificity for the viral enzyme can be achieved with respect to related host cell enzymes [44].

NS4A

NS4A is small (54-amino-acid) HCV protein containing three distinct domains. Its central domain mediates the above-mentioned role as a cofactor for NS3's protease activity. The hydrophobic N-terminal segment is responsible for NS4A's membrane targeting and the recruitment of NS3 to membranes. The acidic C-terminal domain has recently been found to harbor amino acids that are important for establishing RNA replication [45] and that may define an interaction with NS3 that might be targetable by rational drug design. Finally, NS4A may have another function in the context of a precursor protein in which NS4A remains linked to NS4B. Expression of this precursor inhibited general ER to Golgi traffic, including the transport of newly synthesized MHC-I to the cell surface [46].

NS4B

NS4B is an HCV NS protein that until recently was characterized mainly by its lack of known function. Individual reports have suggested that NS4B might inhibit translation, modulate NS5B function, recruit other NS proteins into a protected intracellular compartment with characteristics of lipid rafts, or mediate cellular transformation [47–50]. Perhaps most critical for the integrity of the HCV life cycle is NS4B's ability to induce the novel intracellular membrane structures, termed membranous webs, that represent the candidate sites for replication complex assembly (Fig. 4) [51]. NS4B thus seems to play a key role in membrane-associated RNA replication. Attempts to understand the mechanisms underlying its function have led to the identification of new potential targets for drug development.

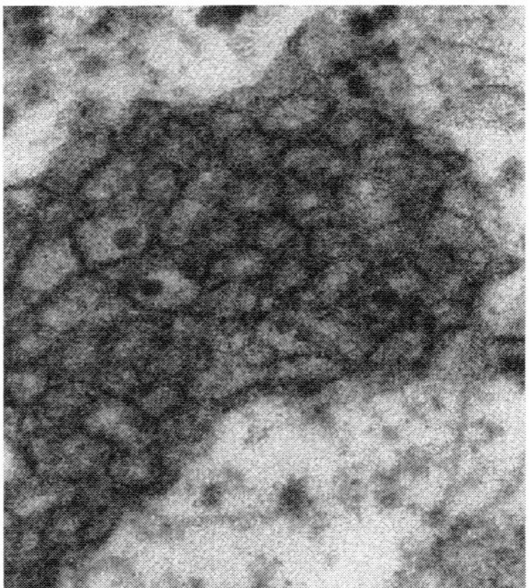

Fig. 4. Electron micrograph of the membranous web. The membranous web is a novel intracellular membrane structure that is induced by HCV and seems to be the platform upon which replication occurs. The viral RNA and individual viral proteins involved in its replication localize to this apparent collection of vesicles clustered together within a web of membranes. The figure is an enlarged segment of a cell harboring the HCV polyprotein.

NS4B is tightly associated with intracellular membranes, and several predicted transmembrane domains have been proposed to account for this [52]. NS4B also contains a predicted N-terminal amphipathic helix (Fig. 5) that can mediate membrane association in the absence of all predicted transmembrane domains. Moreover, the NS4B amphipathic helix (AH) seems to help assemble the components of the HCV replication complex, and disrupting the function of this AH abrogates HCV RNA replication [53].

NS4B has recently been shown to harbor a nucleotide binding motif (NBM). This NBM mediates GTP binding and GTPase activity. The GTPase activity seems to be essential for HCV replication [54]. Because the NS4B NBM has some unique features that distinguish it from host cell GTP-binding proteins, it represents an attractive target for drug development. In addition, it may be amenable to small molecule inhibitor design.

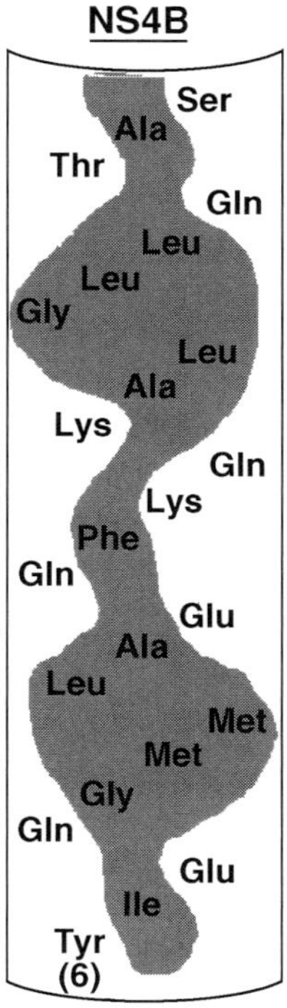

Fig. 5. The N-terminus of NS4B contains an amphipathic alpha helix. This region of NS4B is predicted to adopt an alpha helical secondary structure. It is depicted above in a helix net diagram wherein the cylindrical alpha-helical segment is "cut" longitudinally along one face and then "flattened" into the plane of the page. The amino acid sequence of NS4B from amino acids 6 to 29 in the N-terminal to C-terminal direction is shown. Hydrophobic amino acids in the amphipathic helix are shaded. Note the long, continuous stretch of such amino acids along one face of the helix, defining its amphipathic nature.

NS5A

NS5A has been implicated in interactions with a variety of host cell intracellular signaling and antiviral pathways. A lot of attention has focused on its possible role in modulating the response to IFN treatment. As these interactions become better defined and if they are found to be generalized across HCV infections, they may yield new targets for therapy. A more immediate target has emerged from studies focused on the mechanism of NS5A's membrane association and its role in HCV RNA replication.

All positive-strand RNA viruses studied to date have a common feature of their replication strategy. The RNA-directed RNA replication occurs in association with a specialized subset of intracellular membranes. For some viruses, the latter are pre-existing membrane compartments such as endosomes, whereas other viruses induce novel membrane structures that become their platform for replication. Because this is a feature critical for the virus but not its host cell, this is a promising area for antiviral intervention. Studying the mechanistic details of how HCV induces and maintains its membrane-associated replication complex has begun to identify interesting new potential anti-HCV strategies.

That NS5A might play a role in membrane-associated RNA replication was suggested by the protein's ability to localize to a subset of host cell intracellular membranes. Intriguingly, however, NS5A possesses no classical transmembrane domains to explain how it localizes to membranes. The answer to this puzzle turns out to reside in a small stretch of amino acids near the protein's N-terminus. As found in NS4B, this segment consists of an amphipathic alpha helix. Unlike NS4B, NS5A has no other predicted transmembrane domains to account for its membrane association, and the NS5A amphipathic helix has been proposed to anchor the protein by inserting the hydrophobic face of the helix into the plane of the membrane [55]. If the hydrophobic face is genetically disrupted, NS5A membrane association is lost, and HCV RNA replication is abolished [56]. Pharmacologic inhibitors that can similarly interfere with the ability of the AH to mediate membrane association would offer a new approach to anti-HCV therapy. One type of such inhibitors is a peptide mimic of the NS5A amphipathic helix and is designed to compete with the viral NS5A for its membrane-binding site [56]. Proof-of-concept for another type of peptide inhibitor—one that is a direct ligand of the NS5A amphipathic helix—has been recently obtained (Cheong KH, Smith R, Nolan GP, et al, unpublished observations).

NS5B

NS5B is another target for drug development because its RNA-dependent RNA polymerization activity is a virus-specific feature; our cells are not supposed to have such enzymes, and therefore the potential for selectivity exists. Moreover, like inhibitors of the viral protease, there is precedence for a collection of drugs successfully targeting polymerases in other viruses, such as HBV and HIV. The crystal structure of NS5B has also been solved [57]. It shares several similarities to other viral RNA-dependent RNA polymerases, although it has some unique features. Such detailed knowledge of the protein's structure is invaluable to rational drug design and optimization.

Nucleoside [58,59] and non-nucleosidc inhibitors [60–63] have been developed. Structural and resistance-mapping studies have revealed that current inhibitors fall into two distinct classes: those that directly target the enzyme's active site and those that bind elsewhere on the protein and function as allo-steric inhibitors.

Although NS5B encodes the catalytic activity for RNA polymerization, the overall HCV replication complex is likely composed of other NS proteins as well. Thus, inhibitors developed solely against purified NS5B may prove disappointing when evaluated against actively replicating virus in cells.

Cis-acting elements

Specific sequence elements in the HCV RNA genome are being considered as potential antiviral targets. These so-called "cis-acting elements" include the IRES and conserved RNA structural motifs in the HCV nontranslated regions (NTRs). In addition, at least one cis-acting sequence element has been described within the coding region of NS5B [64]. Because these are RNA targets, antisense and ribozyme-based strategies for drug development have been initiated. siRNA technology [65] may also be suitable for these targets, especially if the RNA targets are accessible enough during the viral replication cycle. Achieving adequate delivery of nucleic acid-based drugs may be the biggest obstacle. Small molecule or peptide ligands of these RNA targets may also be considered.

Host targets

Recent work suggests that prenylation inhibitors may have activity against HCV. Such compounds target the enzyme(s) responsible for attaching post-translational prenyl lipid modifications to proteins. The addition of prenyl lipids—or prenylation—is essential for the function of a variety of proteins. When added to cells harboring HCV replicons, the prenylation inhibitor GGTI-286 prevented the formation of HCV replication complexes and RNA replication, although the precise protein whose inhibited prenylation is responsible for this effect was not clarified [66]. This represents an example of a new approach to antiviral therapy [67]. In contrast to classical antivirals that target a virus-specific enzyme, prenylation inhibitors target a host cell enzyme and thereby seek to deprive the virus access to a host cell function. One interesting consequence may be to make the development of resistance a more difficult task because the targeted locus is not under genetic control of the virus.

Individual genes capable of modulating host antiviral mechanisms may yield new targets for drag development. For example, IRF-3 has been shown to be at a key intersection of the virus–host response interface [68]. Drugs designed to promote signaling through the IRF-3 pathway in HCV-infected cells may help stimulate the host antiviral response. Immunomodulatory therapy [69] and the use of growth factors are other areas of potential antiviral development, and the latter is covered in great detail in the article by Curry and Afdhal elsewhere in this issue.

The above approaches and other agents which target host cell functions are not necessarily specific for just HCV. In that sense, they take us partially full circle, sharing features with current first-generation agents.

Hepatitis C virus replicons

When considering efforts aimed at better understanding the HCV life cycle and the identification of targets for drug development, it is imperative to at least briefly review the development of HCV replicons. The latter represent one of the most important advances since the first cloning of the virus and are becoming a standard feature of research in the field.

The study of HCV replication has been hampered by the lack of a convenient cell culture system. A major problem has been that neither virus isolated from serum nor in vitro-transcribed RNA corresponding to the full-length genome is capable of initiating efficient replication in cultured cells. The first breakthrough was provided by Lohman and colleagues [35]. They constructed a bicistronic RNA molecule derived from HCV in which the virus' structural genes were removed and replaced with a drug resistance gene (neomycinphosphotransferase, or "neo," which confers resistance to the drug G418) (Fig. 6). This so-called "subgenomic HCV replicon" (Fig. 6B) contains the HCV NS proteins thought to constitute the viral replication machinery and the conserved 5′and 3′ NTR regions at the ends of the HCV genomic RNA, which are presumed recognition sequences for the viral replication complex. Delivery of such a replicon to the human liver tumor-derived Huh-7 cell line, followed by selection in G418, led to colonies composed of individual cells each harboring replicating replicons that provided enough neomycin resistance to allow growth in the presence of the selecting drug, G418. The efficiency of colony formation was quite low, approximately one colony for every 10^6 electroporated cells (Fig. 7A). This was sufficient, however, to permit the next important advancement.

Formally, the colonies obtained in such assays could result from a mutation in the host Huh-7 cells, which confers resistance to G418 or allows increased replicon replication. An example of the latter has recently been described [70]. Many of the colonies are the result of a mutation that has occurred in the replicon. This was first shown by Blight and colleagues [34], who isolated and sequenced the replicon RNA from individual colonies

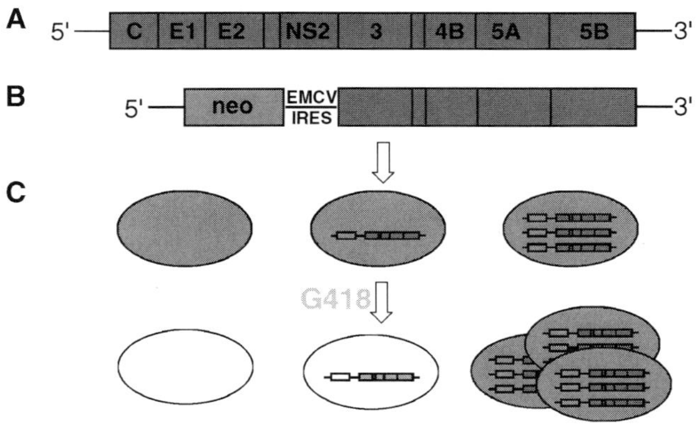

Fig. 6. Schematic of HCV sub-genomic replicons. (*A*) The full-length HCV genome. (*B*) HCV subgenomic replicon in which the HCV structural genes have been replaced with the neomycin phosphotransferase gene, which confers resistance to the drug G418 (E-IRES, encephalomyocarditis internal ribosome entry site). (*C*) HCV subgenomic replicons are delivered to Huh-7 cells, and G418 selection is applied. Cells that do not take up replicons or in which the replicons do not replicate (left and middle of figure) die in the presence of G418. Cells in which the replicons do replicate, and thereby provide a source of neomycin phosphotransferase, survive and multiply to yield a colony (right of figure).

and found that specific so-called "adaptive" mutations had occurred that allowed the replicons to replicate with much greater efficiency. By incorporating selected adaptive mutations into the original replicon of Lohman and colleagues [35] and repeating the original experiment, they observed up to

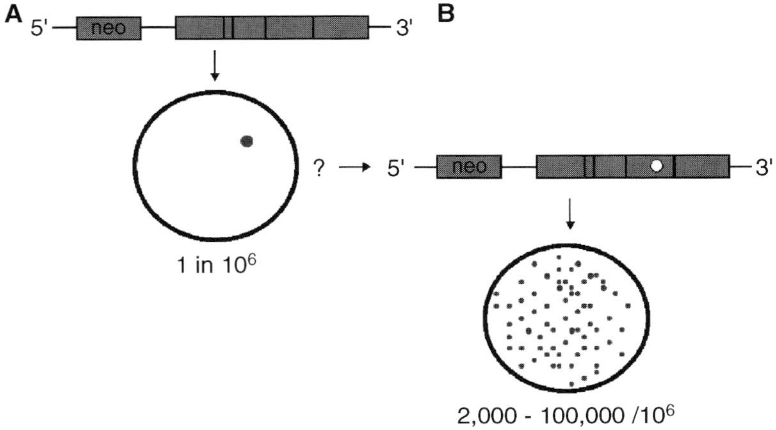

Fig. 7. Isolation of high-efficiency HCV subgenomic replicons. (*A*) The original HCV replicon from Lohman and colleagues [35] was delivered to Huh-7 cells, and G418 selection was applied. Rare colonies were obtained. (*B*) Sequencing of the replicons in the colony reveals a new mutation (*white dot*). The new mutation is incorporated into a new stock of HCV replicons, and the experiment is repeated. This time, colony formation efficiency is increased by 4 logs [34].

4 logs increase in colony formation efficiency [34] (Fig. 7B). Although they are not a complete substitute for a culture system permitting infection with natural HCV virions, these second-generation, high-efficiency replicons are an important breakthrough. They open the prospect of performing detailed molecular genetic studies and are ideal for the evaluation of candidate drugs. An example of such genetic studies is shown in Fig. 8, where the effect of disrupting the amphipathic helix of NS5A is tested. A replicon harboring a mutated amphipathic helix (Fig. 8B) is compared with a wild-type replicon (Fig. 8A). The dramatic effect of such mutation is readily apparent by the lack of colonies on the mutant plate. One can imagine how a drug with potential anti-HCV activity can be assayed in such a system.

Recent improvements in replicon technology include the incorporation of the coding region of the structural proteins to yield so-called "full-length" replicons [71] and the expansion of the range of host cells capable of harboring HCV replicons [72,73]. Finally, the recent reports of full-length genomes capable of generating secreted HCV particles which can re-infect cells represent a potentially dramatic breakthrough, as they should enable an array of exciting new research and drug development [74–76].

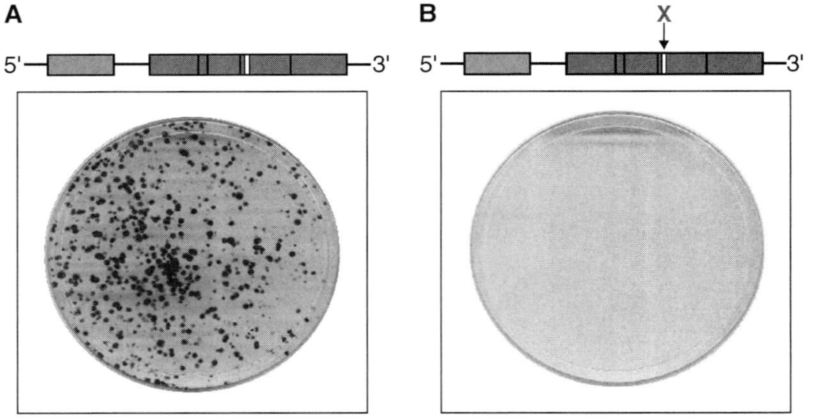

Fig. 8. Effect of disrupting the NS5A amphipathic helix on HCV RNA replication. (*A*) A wild-type, high-efficiency HCV replicon (diagrammed at the top of the figure) was delivered to Huh-7 cells, and G418 selection was applied in a standard colony formation assay, the basis of which is outlined in Figs. 6 and 7. The plate was stained with cresyl violet to reveal the presence of colonies. Numerous colonies were obtained, indicating good HCV genome replication (*lower panel*). (*B*) A mutant replicon (diagrammed at the top of the figure) was constructed by introducing mutations (indicated by "X") into the region of the high-efficiency HCV replicon, which encodes for the hydrophobic face of the NS5A amphipathic helix. This mutant replicon was subjected to the same type of colony formation assay as in (*A*). As shown in the lower panel, no colonies were obtained, indicating that HCV RNA replication was abrogated (*lower panel*). These results genetically validate the NS5A amphipathic helix as a potential new antiviral target (see Ref. [56] for additional details).

Summary

With the advent of second-generation agents that for the first time specifically target individual HCV proteins, HCV-specific therapy has arrived. The study of HCV molecular virology has helped make this possible and is helping us to identify additional new antiviral targets that will be targeted by third-generation drugs. Key to these efforts is the development of high-efficiency HCV replicons. The future effective pharmacologic control of HCV will likely consist of a cocktail of simultaneously administered virus-specific agents with independent targets. This should minimize the emergence of resistance against any single agent. The way we treat HCV should change dramatically over the next few years.

Acknowledgments

This work was supported in part by R01-DK066793, R01-DK064223, a Burroughs Wellcome Fund Career Development Award, and a Burroughs Wellcome Fund Clinical Scientist Award in Translational Research.

References

[1] Alter MJ, Kruszon-Moran D, Nainan OV, et al. The prevalence of Hepatitis C virus infection in the United States, 1988 through 1994. New Engl Med J 1999;341:556–62.
[2] Di Bisceglie AM. Natural history of hepatitis C: its impact on clinical management. Hepatology 2000;31:1014–8.
[3] McHutchison JG, Gordon SC, Schiff ER, et al. Interferon alfa-2b alone or in combination with ribavirin as initial treatment for chronic hepatitis C. Hepatitis Interventional Therapy Group. N Engl J Med 1998;339:1485–92.
[4] Liang TJ, Rehermann B, Seeff LB, et al. Pathogenesis, natural history, treatment, and prevention of hepatitis C. Ann Intern Med 2000;132:296–305.
[5] Zeuzem S, Feinman SV, Rasenack J, et al. Peginterferon alfa-2a in patients with chronic hepatitis C. N Engl J Med 2000;343:1666–72.
[6] Bartenschlager R, Lohmann V. Replication of hepatitis C virus. J Gen Virol 2000;81:1631–48.
[7] Branch AD. Hepatitis C virus RNA codes for proteins and replicates: does it also trigger the interferon response? Semin Liver Dis 2000;20:57–68.
[8] Reed KE, Rice CM. Overview of hepatitis C virus genome structure, polyprotein processing, and protein properties. Curr Top Microbiol Immunol 2000;242:55–84.
[9] Agnello V, Abel G, Elfahal M, et al. Hepatitis C virus and other flaviviridae viruses enter cells via low density lipoprotein receptor. Proc Natl Acad Sci USA 1999;96:I2766–71.
[10] Cormier EG, Durso RJ, Tsamis F, et al. L-SIGN (CD209L) and DC-SIGN (CD209) mediate transinfection of liver cells by hepatitis C virus. Proc Natl Acad Sci USA 2004;101:14067–72.
[11] Pileri P, Uematsu Y, Campagnoli S, et al. Binding of hepatitis C virus to CD81. Science 1998;282:938–41.
[12] Scarselli E, Ansuini H, Cerino R, et al. The human scavenger receptor class B type I is a novel candidate receptor for the hepatitis C virus. EMBO J 2002;21:5017–25.
[13] Gosert R, Egger D, Lohmann V, et al. Identification of the hepatitis C virus RNA replication complex in Huh-7 cells harboring subgenomic replicons. J Virol 2003;77:5487–92.

[14] Ray RB, Meyer K, Ray R. Suppression of apoptotic cell death by hepatitis C virus core protein. Virology 1996;226:176–82.
[15] Watashi K, Hijikata M, Tagawa A, et al. Modulation of retinoid signaling by a cytoplasmic viral protein via sequestration of Sp110b, a potent transcriptional corepressor of retinoic acid receptor, from the nucleus. Mol Cell Biol 2003;23:7498–509.
[16] Ohkawa K, Ishida H, Nakanishi F, et al. Hepatitis C virus core functions as a suppressor of cyclin-dependent kinase-activating kinase and impairs cell cycle progression. J Biol Chem 2004;279:11719–26.
[17] Hosui A, Ohkawa K, Ishida H, et al. Hepatitis C virus core protein differently regulates the JAK-STAT signaling pathway under interleukin-6 and interferon-gamma stimuli. J Biol Chem 2003;278:28562–7.
[18] Zhu N, Khoshnan A, Schneider R, et al. Hepatitis C virus core protein binds to the cytoplasmic domain of tumor necrosis factor (TNF) receptor 1 and enhances TNF-induced apoptosis. J Virol 1998;72:3691–7.
[19] Kunkel M, Lorinczi M, Rijnbrand R, et al. Self-assembly of nucleocapsid-like particles from recombinant hepatitis C virus core protein. J Virol 2001;75:2119–29.
[20] Acosta-Rivero N, Rodriguez A, Musacchio A, et al. In vitro assembly into virus-like particles is an intrinsic quality of Pichia pastoris derived HCV core protein. Biochem Biophys Res Commun 2004;325:68–74.
[21] Deres K, Schroder CH, Paessens A, et al. Inhibition of hepatitis B virus replication by drug-induced depletion of nucleocapsids. Science 2003;299:893–6.
[22] Chazal N, Gerlier D. Virus entry, assembly, budding, and membrane rafts. Microbiol Mol Biol Rev 2003;67:226–37.
[23] Matto M, Rice CM, Aroeti B, et al. Hepatitis C virus core protein associates with detergent-resistant membranes distinct from classical plasma membrane rafts. J Virol 2004;78: 12047–53.
[24] Walewski JL, Keller TR, Stump DD, et al. Evidence for a new hepatitis C virus antigen encoded in an overlapping reading frame. RNA 2001;7:710–21.
[25] Xu Z, Choi J, Yen TS, et al. Synthesis of a novel hepatitis C virus protein by ribosomal frameshift. EMBO J 2001;20:3840–8.
[26] Bain C, Parroche P, Lavergne JP, et al. Memory T-cell-mediated immune responses specific to an alternative core protein in hepatitis C virus infection. J Virol 2004;78:10460–9.
[27] Dubuisson J, Hsu HH, Cheung RC, et al. Formation and intracelluiar localization of hepatitis C virus envelope glycoprotein complexes expressed by recombinant vaccinia and Sindbis viruses. J Virol 1994;68:6147–60.
[28] Santolini E, Migliaccio G, La Monica N. Biosynthesis and biochemical properties of the hepatitis C virus core protein. J Virol 1994;68:3631–41.
[29] Cocquerel L, Op de Beeck A, Lambot M, et al. Topological changes in the transmembrane domains of hepatitis C virus envelope glycoproteins. EMBO J 2002;21:2893–902.
[30] Bartosch B, Dubuisson J, Cosset FL. Infectious hepatitis C virus pseudo-particles containing functional E1–E2 envelope protein complexes. J Exp Med 2003;197:633–42.
[31] Griffin SD, Beales LP, Clarke DS, et al. The p7 protein of hepatitis C virus forms an ion channel that is blocked by the antiviral drug, Amantadine. FEBS Lett 2003;535: 34–8.
[32] Sakai A, Claire MS, Faulk K, et al. The p7 polypeptide of hepatitis C virus is critical for infectivity and contains functionally important genotype-specific sequences. Proc Natl Acad Sci USA 2003;100:11646–51.
[33] Pieroni L, Santolini E, Fipaldini C, et al. In vitro study of the NS2–3 protease of hepatitis C virus. J Virol 1997;71:6373–80.
[34] Blight KJ, Kolykhalov A, Rice CM. Efficient initiation of HCV RNA replication in cell culture. Science 2001;290:1972–4.
[35] Lohmann V, Korner F, Koch J, et al. Replication of subgenomic hepatitis C virus RNAs in a hepatoma cell line. Science 1999;285:110–3.

[36] Kim JL, Morgenstern KA, Lin C, et al. Crystal structure of the hepatitis C virus NS3 protease domain complexed with a synthetic NS4A cofactor peptide. Cell 1996;87:343–55.
[37] Love RA, Parge HE, Wickersham JA, et al. The crystal structure of hepatitis C virus NS3 proteinase reveals a trypsin-like fold and a structural zinc binding site. Cell 1996;87:331–42.
[38] Yao N, Reichert P, Taremi SS, et al. Molecular views of viral ployprotein processing revealed by the crystal structure of the hepatitis C virus bifunctional protease-helicase. Struct Fold Des 1999;7:1353–63.
[39] Kim JL, Morgenstern KA, Griffith JP, et al. Hepatitis C virus NS3 RNA helicase domain with a bound oligonucleotide: the crystal structure provides insights into the mode of unwinding. Structure 1998;6:89–100.
[40] Lamarre D, Anderson PC, Bailey M, et al. An NS3 protease inhibitor with antiviral effects in humans infected with hepatitis C virus. Nature 2003;426:186–9.
[41] Hinrichsen H, Benhamou Y, Wedemeyer H, et al. Short-term antiviral efficacy of BILN 2061, a hepatitis C virus serine protease inhibitor, in hepatitis C genotype 1 patients. Gastroenterology 2004;127:1347–55.
[42] Perni RB, Pitlik J, Britt SD, et al. Inhibitors of hepatitis C virus NS3.4A protease 2: warhead SAR and optimization. Bioorg Med Chem Lett 2004;14:1441–6.
[43] Borowski P, Deinert J, Schalinski S, et al. Halogenated benzimidazoles and benzotriazoles as inhibitors of the NTPase/helicase activities of hepatitis C and related viruses. Bur J Biochem 2003;270:1645–53.
[44] Kim JW, Seo MY, Shelat A, et al. Structurally conserved amino Acid w501 is required for RNA helicase activity but is not essential for DNA helicase activity of hepatitis C virus NS3 protein. J Virol 2003;77:571–82.
[45] Lindenbach BD, Pragai BM, Rice CM. 2004. The C-terminal acidic domain of HCV NS4A is a critical determinant of replication. In: 11th International Symposium on HCV & Related Viruses. Heidelberg: 2004. p. 25.
[46] Konan KV, Giddings TH Jr, Ikeda M, et al. Nonstructural protein precursor NS4A/B from hepatitis C virus alters function and ultrastructure of host secretory apparatus. J Virol 2003; 77:7843–55.
[47] Florese RH, Nagano-Fujii M, Iwanaga Y, et al. Inhibition of protein synthesis by the nonstructural proteins NS4A and NS4B of hepatitis C virus. Virus Res 2002;90:119–31.
[48] Piccininni S, Varaklioti A, Nardelli M, et al. Modulation of the hepatitis C virus RNA-dependent RNA polymerase activity by the non-structural (NS) 3 helicase and the NS4B membrane protein. J Biol Chem 2002;277:45670–9.
[49] Gao L, Aizaki H, He JW, et al. Interactions between viral nonstructural proteins and host protein hVAP-33 mediate the formation of hepatitis C virus RNA replication complex on lipid raft. J Virol 2004;78:3480–8.
[50] Park IS, Yang JM, Min MK. Hepatitis C virus nonstructural protein NS4B transforms NIH3T3 cells in cooperation with the Ha-ras oncogene. Biochem Biophys Res Commun 2000;267:581–7.
[51] Gosert R, Egger D, Lohmann V, et al. Identification of the hepatitis C virus RNA replication complex in Huh-7 cells harboring subgenomic replicons. J Virol 2003;77:5487–92.
[52] Lundin M, Monne M, Widell A, et al. Topology of the membrane-associated hepatitis C virus protein NS4B. J Virol 2003;77:5428–38.
[53] Elazar M, Liu P, Rice CM, et al. Au N-terminal amphipathic helix in hepatitis C virus (HCV) NS4B mediates membrane association, correct localization of replication complex proteins, and HCV RNA replication. J Virol 2004;78:11393–400.
[54] Einav S, Elazar M, Danieli T, et al. A nucleotide binding motif in hepatitis C virus (HCV) NS4B mediates HCV RNA replication. J Virol 2004;78:11288–95.
[55] Penin F, Brass V, Appel N, et al. Structure and function of the membrane anchor domain of hepatitis C virus nonstructural protein 5A. J Biol Chem 2004;279:40835–43.
[56] Elazar M, Cheong KH, Liu P, et al. Amphipathic helix-dependent localization of NS5A mediates hepatitis C virus RNA replication. J Virol 2003;77:6055–61.

[57] Lesburg CA, Cable MB, Ferrari E, et al. Crystal structure of the RNA-dependent RNA polymerase from hepatitis C virus reveals a fully encircled active site. Nat Struct Biol 1999;6:937–43.
[58] Shim J, Larson G, Lai V, et al. Canonical 3′-deoxyribonucleotides as a chain terminator for HCV NS5B RNA-dependent RNA polymerase. Antiviral Res 2003;58:243–51.
[59] Eldrup AB, Prhavc M, Brooks J, et al. Structure-activity relationship of heterobase-modified 2′-C-methyl ribonucleosides as inhibitors of hepatitis C virus RNA replication. J Med Chem 2004;47:5284–97.
[60] Beaulieu PL, Bos M, Bousquet Y, et al. Non-nucleoside inhibitors of the hepatitis C virus NS5B polymerase: discovery of benzimidazole 5-carboxylic amide derivatives with low-nanomolar potency. Bioorg Med Chem Lett 2004;14:967–71.
[61] Chan L, Pereira O, Reddy TJ, et al. Discovery of thiophene-2-carboxylic acids as potent inhibitors of HCV NS5B polymerase and HCV subgenomic RNA replication. Part 2: tertiary amides. Bioorg Med Chem Lett 2004;14:797–800.
[62] Chan L, Das SK, Reddy TJ, et al. Discovery of thiophene-2-carboxylic acids as potent inhibitors of HCV NS5B polymerase and HCV subgenomic RNA replication. Part 1: sulfonamides. Bioorg Med Chem Lett 2004;14:793–6.
[63] Gu B, Johnston VK, Gutshall LL, et al. Arresting initiation of hepatitis C virus RNA synthesis using heterocyclic derivatives. J Biol Chem 2003;278:16602–7.
[64] You S, Stump DD, Branch AD, et al. A cis-acting replication element in the sequence encoding the NS5B RNA-dependent RNA polymerase is required for hepatitis C virus RNA replication. J Virol 2004;78:1352–66.
[65] Radhakrishnan SK, Layden TJ, Cartel AL. RNA interference as a new strategy against viral hepatitis. Virology 2004;323:173–81.
[66] Ye J, Wang C, Sumpter R Jr, et al. Disruption of hepatitis C virus RNA replication through inhibition of host protein geranylgeranylation. Proc Natl Acad Sci USA 2003;100:15865–70.
[67] Einav S, Glenn JS. Prenylation inhibitors: a novel class of antiviral agents. J Antimicrob Chemother 2003;52:883–6.
[68] Foy E, Li K, Wang C, et al. Regulation of interferon regulatory factor-3 by the hepatitis C virus serine protease. Science 2003;300:1145–8.
[69] McHutchison JG, Dev AT. Future trends in managing hepatitis C. Gastroenterol Clin North Am 2004;33:S51–61.
[70] Blight KJ, McKeating JA, Rice CM. Highly permissive cell lines for subgenomic and genomic hepatitis C virus RNA replication. J Virol 2002;76:13001–14.
[71] Pietschmann T, Lohmann V, Kaul A, et al. Persistent and transient replication of full-length hepatitis C virus genomes in cell culture. J Virol 2002;76:4008–21.
[72] Zhu Q, Guo JT, Seeger C. Replication of hepatitis C virus subgenomes in nonhepatic epithelial and mouse hepatoma cells. J Virol 2003;77:9204–10.
[73] Kato T, Date T, Miyamoto M, et al. Nonhepatic cell lines HeLa and 293 support efficient replication of the hepatitis c virus genotype 2a subgenomic replicon. J Virol 2005;79:592–6.
[74] Lindenbach BD, Evans MJ, Syder AJ, et al. Complete replication of hepatitis C virus in cell culture. Science 2005;309(5734):623–6.
[75] Zhong J, Gastaminza P, Cheng G, et al. Robust hepatitis C virus infection in vitro. Proc Natl Acad Sci USA 2005;102(26):9294–9.
[76] Wakita T, Pietschmann T, Kato T, et al. Production of infectious hepatitis C virus in tissue culture from a cloned viral genome. Nat Med 2005;11:791–6.

ELSEVIER
SAUNDERS

Infect Dis Clin N Am
20 (2006) 99–113

INFECTIOUS
DISEASE CLINICS
OF NORTH AMERICA

Antiviral Therapy for Treatment Naïve Patients with Hepatitis C Virus

Sangik Oh, MD, MMSc[a,b], Nezam H. Afdhal, MD[a,b,*]

[a]*Department of Medicine, Harvard Medical School, 25 Shattack Street, Boston, MA 02115, USA*

[b]*The Liver Center, Beth Israel Deaconess Medical Center, 110 Francis Street, Suite 8E, Boston, MA 02215, USA*

Chronic hepatitis C virus (HCV) infection is recognized as a global health problem, with 170 to 200 million people estimated to be infected worldwide. In the United States, chronic HCV is the most common cause of end-stage liver disease, hepatocellular cancer, and the most frequent indication for liver transplantation [1]. Data from the third National Health and Nutrition Examination Survey (NHANES III) estimated that 2.7 million Americans have active HCV infection [2]. This figure probably underestimates the true prevalence of chronic HCV infection, however, as the study excluded high-risk groups such as prisoners and homeless people. HCV infection generally is regarded as "a disease of decades," as the most significant clinical consequences occur 20 to 30 years after the initial exposure. Approximately 10,000 HCV related deaths occur each year, mostly resulting from end-stage liver disease and development of hepatocellular carcinoma (HCC) [3]. The NHANES study also revealed that HCV prevalence was the highest in persons 30 to 49 years of age. Because of its slowly progressive natural history, the Centers for Disease Control and Prevention (CDC) predict that HCV-associated mortality might double or triple over the next 10 to 20 years [4]. Davis et al estimated that the need for liver transplantation will increase by 528%, and liver-related death might increase by 223% by 2008 [5]. One logical solution is early detection and aggressive antiviral treatment to eradicate HCV or to halt disease progression.

A version of this article originally appeared in the 33:3 issue of Gastroenterology Clinics of North America.

* Corresponding author.

E-mail address: nafdhal@bidmc.harvard.edu (N.H. Afdhal).

0891-5520/06/$ - see front matter
doi:10.1016/j.idc.2006.01.007 *id.theclinics.com*

This article focuses on the most recent therapies for patients with HCV who are naïve to therapy. The primary end point for the treatment of naïve HCV patients is viral eradication or a sustained virological response (SVR), which is defined as the absence of HCV in the serum, as detected by a sensitive polymerase chain reaction (PCR) test, 24 weeks after stopping antiviral therapy. Recent data suggest that an SVR can be equated with a biochemical, virological, and histological response that is sustained for up to 5 years and is conceptually a cure of HCV in 90% of patients [6]. Some patients fail to clear HCV by PCR while on treatment, and these are classified as nonresponders (NR). Additionally, there is a final group of relapsers, who are able to clear HCV on treatment, but in whom HCV reappears within 24 weeks of stopping treatment. These definitions of patient responses are used in the clinical trials discussed in this article.

Patient selection

The indications for therapy for naïve patients have undergone many revisions over the last 10 years (Box 1). Patients who are HCV-positive by PCR test with an elevated alanine aminotransferase (ALT) and necro-

Box 1. Indications and contraindications to therapy

Indications
Elevated/normal ALT
Necro-inflammation and fibrosis on liver biopsy
Hepatitis C virus RNA positive
Extrahepatic manifestations (renal disease, cryoglobulinemia, porphyria cutanea tarda)
Patient preference

Contraindications
Absolute
Severe uncontrolled depression
Unstable cardiac disease
Uncontrolled concomitant disease
Pregnancy
Hemolytic diseases
Renal disease; creatinine greater than 2 mg/dL
Seizure disorder
Relative
Active drug and alcohol use
Moderate depression/situational suicidal ideation
Decompensated liver disease
Autoimmune diseases

inflammation and fibrosis on liver biopsy are obvious candidates for treatment. At the National Institutes of Health (NIH) consensus conference in 2002, however, there was a strong movement toward expanding the number of potential treatment candidates to include people with controlled depressive illness, methadone users, and patients who had stopped using alcohol recently. The other controversial area is whether to treat patients with persistently normal ALT. In the era of interferon (IFN) monotherapy, several case series suggested that patients with normal ALT might experience ALT flares and have a reduced SVR rate if treated with IFN [7,8]. Larger studies with IFN and ribavirin (RBV), however, have shown that ALT flares are not common and that the SVR rate is similar in patients with normal ALT compared with those with elevated ALT [9,10]. The current recommendation is that treatment of patients with normal ALT be considered on an individual basis, and it is believed that these patients will respond equally well to IFN and RBV combination therapy.

There remain some absolute contraindications to treatment, and these are listed in Box 1. In particular, therapy should not be undertaken in patients with decompensated liver disease and with active manic depressive disease or recent suicidal ideation. RBV is contraindicated specifically in patients with hemolytic disease, unstable cardiac disease, renal disease with a creatinine above 2.0 mg/dL, and in patients who are pregnant or contemplating pregnancy.

Historical perspective

The efficacy of alpha interferon for treatment of HCV first was recognized when Hoofnagle et al published their preliminary findings in 1986 when HCV was known as non-A, non-B hepatitis [11]. They treated 10 patients with chronic non-A, non-B hepatitis with varying doses (0.5 to 5 million U) up to 12 months. The aminotransferases levels improved in 8 of 10 patients and in 3 patients who had follow-up biopsies done after 1 year of therapy showing marked improvement in liver histology. Several subsequent studies, including a large, multi-center, randomized clinical trial in the United States by Davis et al confirmed the initial finding that long-term IFN therapy improved liver function tests and liver histology [12]. The US Food and Drug Administration (FDA) approved alpha interferon monotherapy for the treatment of chronic HCV infection in 1993. In 1997, The NIH released the consensus statement recommending alpha interferon monotherapy at a dose of 3 million U three times weekly for 48 weeks as the standard of care for patients with chronic HCV infection. There are three IFNs approved for monotherapy in the United States, including IFN alfa 2b, IFN alfa 2a, and consensus IFN (CIFN). Multiple clinical trials of IFN monotherapy have been published using different doses and schedules, and overall there have been no major clinical differences in SVR between the different IFNs. Overall, the rates of SVR have been limited to 6% to 16%.

The optimal duration of treatment is 48 weeks for IFN monotherapy. In view of this relatively low response rate, higher doses, longer duration, induction doses, and dose escalation have been tried to increase SVR, but none of these variations has been shown prospectively to significantly increase response.

Combination therapy of interferon with ribavirin

A major advance occurred when IFN was combined with RBV in the pivotal studies of McHutchison et al [13], and SVR was increased from 13% to 38%. RBV is a nucleoside analog that putatively acts by means of inhibition of RNA-dependent RNA polymerase, depletion of intracellular guanosine triphosphate pools, and by altering Th1 and Th2 cytokine balance in the liver. Initial studies of RBV monotherapy in HCV resulted in biochemical but not histological response [14–16]. Two large randomized controlled clinical trials comparing IFN/RBV combination therapy with IFN monotherapy in HCV infection demonstrated a significant improvement in SVR for combination therapy (Fig. 1) [13,17]. Combination IFN/RBV therapy became the standard of care for naïve patients, with a 24-week course of

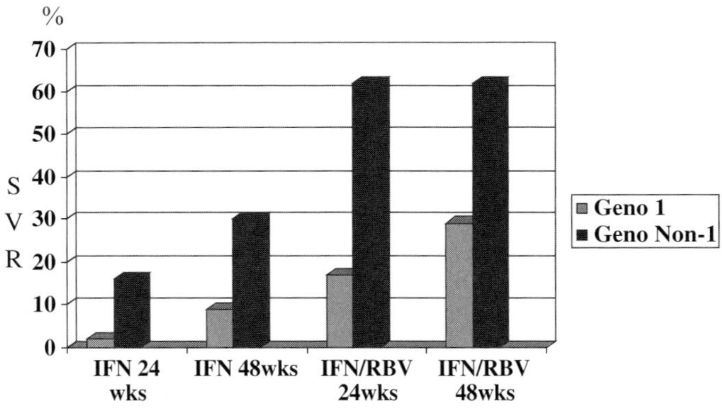

Fig. 1. SVR rates according to genotype for naïve patients receiving IFN alfa-2b versus combination IFN alfa-2b plus 1000/1200 mg ribavirin daily. In genotype non-1 patients, 24 weeks of combination IFN/RBV was equivalent to 48 weeks with a 62% SVR. For genotype 1 patients, SVR was 29% with 48 weeks of combination therapy (*P* less than 0.008 compared with IFN monotherapy for 48 weeks). (*Data from* McHutchison JG, Gordon SC, Schiff ER, Shiffman ML, Lee WM, Rustgi VK, et al. Interferon alfa-2b alone or in combination with ribavirin as initial treatment for chronic hepatitis C. Hepatitis Interventional Therapy Group. N Engl J Med 1998;339(21):1485–92; Poynard T, Marcellin P, Lee SS, Niederau C, Minuk GS, Ideo G, et al. Randomised trial of interferon alfa-2b plus ribavirin for 48 weeks or for 24 weeks versus interferon alfa-2b plus placebo for 48 weeks for treatment of chronic infection with hepatitis C virus. International Hepatitis Interventional Therapy Group (IHIT). Lancet 1998; 352(9138):1426–32.)

treatment for genotyped 2 and 3 patients and a 48-week course for genotype 1 patients.

Pegylated alfa interferon monotherapy

Pegylation is a process by which a polyethylene glycol molecule is attached to a protein or drug to decrease renal clearance and increase bioavailability and efficacy. The renal clearance and short half-life of alfa interferons necessitated their administration three times a week and made them an excellent target molecule for pegylation. A critical concept with pegylation of biologically active proteins is the need to achieve a balance between increasing the half-life while maintaining biological activity. Increasing the size of the pegylated component can decrease renal clearance but also reduces the biological activity of the IFN component. There are two forms of peginterferons that have been approved by the FDA for use in chronic HCV; PEG-IFN 2a (Pegasys) IFN and PEG-IFN 2b (PEG-INTRON). PEG-IFN 2a has a 40kDa branched chain PEG attached to IFN alfa 2a, and PEG-IFN 2b has a 12kDa straight chain PEG attached to IFN alfa 2b. Both PEG-IFNs retain reduced but effective biological activity while having a favorable pharmacological profile that allows for once weekly administration. These PEG-IFNs have replaced IFN as the preferred form of IFN for use in treatment of HCV infection.

Clinical trials have confirmed a twofold increase in efficacy of PEG-IFNs compared with standard IFN in HCV treatment-naïve patients (Table 1). Zeuzem et al showed that in the SVR was 39% in patients treated with PEG-IFN 2a at a dose of 180 μg for 48 weeks compared with 19% in patients taking standard interferon 2a at a dose of 6 mU three times weekly for 12 weeks then 3 mU three times weekly for 36 weeks [18]. In this trial, 62% of the subjects had genotype 1 HCV, and 7% had cirrhosis. In their multivariate analysis, use of PEG-IFN 2a, younger age, smaller body surface area, absence of cirrhosis or bridging fibrosis, a lower HCV RNA level, and a nongenotype 1 infection were associated with higher SVR. Subsequent studies using PEG-IFN 2a have shown a somewhat reduced SVR of 29%.

The results are similar in a study from Lindsay et al comparing there doses of PEG-IFN 2b (0.5, 1.0 and 1.5 μg/kg per week) with standard IFN alfa 2b at 3 mU three times weekly for 48 weeks [19]. The SVR was only 12% with standard IFN but 18%, 25%, and 23%, respectively with escalating doses of PEG-IFN 2b. In this study, two pretreatment variables were associated with higher SVR when a multivariate analysis was performed: nongenotype 1 and HCV RNA less than 2 million copies/mL.

In a difficult-to-treat population of naïve patients with advanced fibrosis, defined as bridging fibrosis or cirrhosis, PEG-IFN 2a again demonstrated superior SVR compared with IFN alfa 2a. Heathcote et al randomized 271 patients with cirrhosis or bridging fibrosis into one of three groups: standard IFN alpha-2a at a dose of 3 mU three times weekly; PEG-IFN

Table 1
Randomized controlled trials of peginterferon monotherapy

Study	Zeuzem et al, 2000		Heathcote et al, 2000			Lindsay et al, 2001			
Type of IFN	IFN a-2a	PegIFN a-2a	IFN a-2a	PegIFN a-2a	PegIFN a-2a	IFN a-2b	PegIFN a-2b	PegIFN a-2b	PegIFN a-2b
Dose and duration	6 mU for 12 weeks, then 3 mU for 36 weeks	180 μg for 48 weeks	3 mU for 48 weeks	90 μg for 48 weeks	180 μg for 48 weeks	3 mU for 48 weeks	0.5 μg/kg/wk	1.0 μg/kg/wk	1.5 μg/kg/wk
Number of patients	264	267	88	96	87	303	315	297	304
Sustained virological response (95% CI)	19% (14 to 24%)	39% (33% to 45%)	7% (4 to 16%)	15% (9 to 23%)	30% (21% to 40%)	12% (9% to 16%)	18% (14% to 23%)	25% (20 to 30%)	23% (19% to 28%)

2a at a dose of 90 μg; and PEG-IFN 2a at a dose of 180 μg for 48 weeks [20]. The SVR was 30% with PEG-IFN 2a at 180 μg compared with 8% for standard IFN alfa 2a.

In summary, the pegylation of interferons has resulted in improving the pharmacokinetic (PK) profile, allowing for once weekly administration while improving the biological activity and doubling the SVR rates for IFN alfa 2a and 2b.

Pegylated interferon and ribavirin combination therapy

A logical extension of the PEG-IFN monotherapy trials was to combine PEG-IFN with RBV, and two large prospective studies have compared combination PEG-IFN/RBV with IFN/RBV. Both trials have demonstrated a significant benefit of the PEG-IFN/RBV combination over standard combination therapy, and PEG-IFN/RBV is the standard of care for naïve chronic HCV patients currently.

Manns et al conducted a randomized clinical trial with PEG-IFN 2b involving 1530 HCV patients from Europe, North America, and Australia [21]. They were randomized into one of three groups: IFN alfa 2b (3 mU three times weekly) with RBV (1000 to 1200 mg daily based on body weight) for 48 weeks, PEG-IFN alfa-2b at 1.5 μg/kg/week with RBV 800 mg daily for 48 weeks, or PEG-IFN alfa-2b at 1.5 μg/kg/week for 4 weeks and then 0.5 μg/kg/week for 44 weeks with standard doses of RBV. The group receiving highest dose of PEG-IFN alfa-2b with RBV achieved highest rate of SVR (54%) when compared with the group that received lower dose of PEG-IFN (47%) and standard IFN (47%) combined with RBV (Table 2).

Fried et al conducted a comparable study with PEG-IFN alfa-2a in combination with RBV [22]. A total of 1121 patients were assigned randomly to one of three groups: standard IFN alfa-2b (3 mU three times weekly) with RBV (1000 to 1200 mg daily based on body weight), PEG-IFN alfa-2a (180 μg weekly) with RBV (1000 to 1200 mg daily based on body weight), or

Table 2
Results from the two clinical trials of peg-interferon and ribavirin

Study	Manns et al 2001			Fried et al 2002		
Interferon Regimen	INF a-2b 3 mU tiw	PegIFN a-2b 1.5 μg/kg/wk	PegIFN 1.5 μg/kg/wk	IFN a-2b 3 mU tiw	PegIFN a-2a 180 μg	PegIFN a-2a 180 μg
Ribavirin	1000 or 1200 mg	1000 or 1200 mg	800 mg	1000 or 1200 mg	Placebo	1000 or 1200 mg
Number of patients	505	514	511	444	224	453
Sustained viral response (95% CI)	47% (42 to 51%)	47% (43% to 52%)	54% (49% to 58%)	44% (40% to 49%)	29% (24% to 36%)	56% (52% to 61%)

Abbreviation: tiw, three times weekly.

PEG-IFN alfa-2a (180 μg weekly) with placebo. All patients were treated for 48 weeks. The SVR was the highest in the group that received PEG-IFN in combination with RBV (56%) compared with IFN alfa 2b and RBV (45%) and PEG-IFN alfa 2a alone (30%) (Table 2).

A third large randomized controlled study has been performed by Hadziyannis et al [23]. The study design was to examine the effect of duration of therapy (24 versus 48 weeks) and of RBV dose (800 mg versus 1000 or 1200 mg) on SVR using fixed-dose PEG-IFN alfa 2a. A total of 1284 patients were stratified, based on their genotype and pretreatment viral load, and randomized into one of four groups: PEG-IFN alfa-2a (180 μg weekly) and RBV at 800 mg daily for 24 weeks, PEG-IFN alfa-2a (180 μg weekly) and RBV at 1000 or 1200 mg daily for 24 weeks, PEG-IFN alfa-2a (180 μg weekly) and RBV at 800 mg daily for 48 weeks or PEG-IFN alfa-2a (180 μg weekly) and RBV at 1000 to 1200 mg daily for 48 weeks. The genotype-specific SVR is shown in Fig. 2 for the four groups. In patients with genotype 1, the highest SVR was obtained in the group that was treated with highest dose of RBV for the longer duration. In contrast, the SVR did not differ significantly among patients with genotypes 2 or 3 regardless of dose of RBV or the duration of therapy. These findings suggest that patients with genotypes 2 and 3 can be treated effectively with PEG-IFN and lower doses of RBV (800 mg) for 24 weeks, whereas patients with genotype 1 should be treated with higher doses of ribavirin (1000 to 1200 mg) for a longer duration.

Pretreatment predictors of response

Analysis of the clinical trials has identified pretreatment predictors of response to PEG-IFN and RBV (Box 2). The major predictor is genotype, with genotype 1 patients having a markedly reduced response (42% to 46%) compared with patients with genotypes 2 and 3 (76% to 82%). After genotype, multiple other factors have lesser predictive value but can still be clinically important when one is individualizing therapy. Clinically relevant predictors that indicate a more difficult-to-treat patient include viral load greater than 2 million by PCR test, presence of advanced fibrosis or cirrhosis, high body mass index, and African American race. Posthoc analysis of the clinical trials has suggested that PEG-IFN alfa 2b, which is dosed on a weight basis at 1.5 μg per kg, may be more effective in patients with a body weight of greater than 75 kg. Similar analyses have suggested that PEG-IFN alfa 2a may be better for genotype 1 patients with high viral load. All analyses suggest that a weight-based dose of RBV should be used for genotype 1 patients, and the authors recommend 12 to 15 mg of RBV per kilogram.

Early virological response

Although useful, the baseline predictors highlighted are a general guideline for discussion with patients as to the likelihood of response to

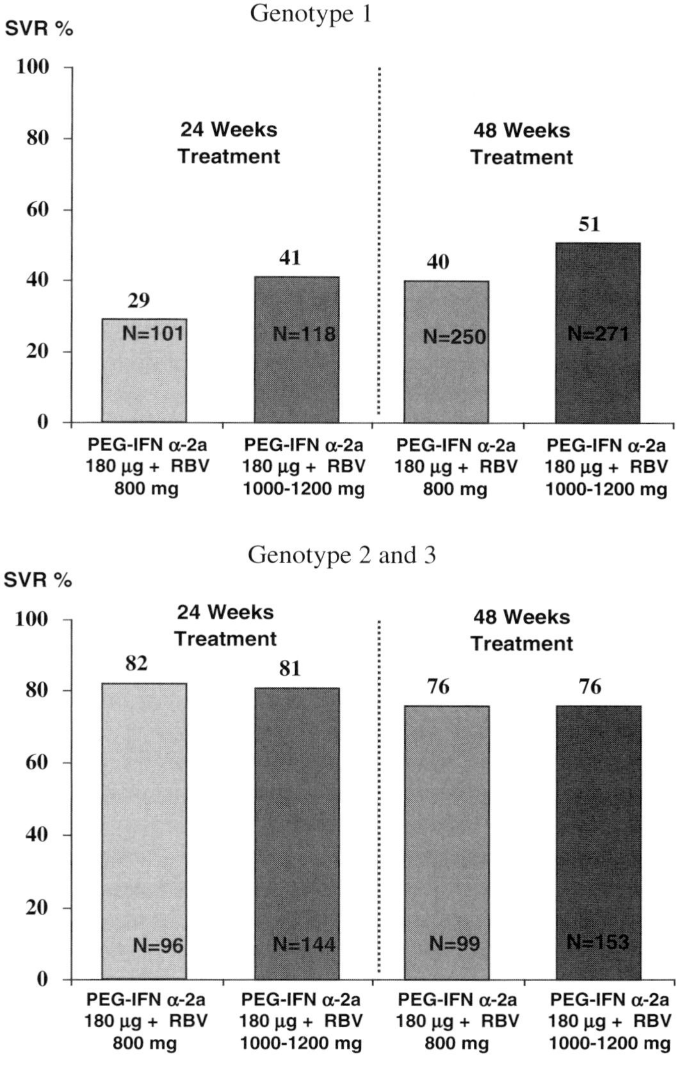

Fig. 2. SVR for four different treatment regimens of PEG-IFN alfa-2a with either RBV 800 mg or 1000/1200 mg given for 24 or 48 weeks. Optimal SVR for genotype 1 is seen with 48 weeks treatment with RBV 1000/1200mg daily. For genotypes 2 and 3, 24 weeks with 800 mg of RBV are equivalent to longer duration of therapy and higher RBV doses. (*Data from* Hadziyannis SJ, Cheinquer H, Morgan T, Diago M, Jensen DM, Sette H. Peginterferon alfa 2-a (40kD) (PEGASYS) in combination with ribavirin (RBV): efficacy and safety results from a phase III randomized double-blind multi-centre study examining effect of duration of treatment and RBV dose. J Hepatol 2002;36(Suppl 1):3.)

Box 2. Factors predicting increased SVR

Fixed

- Genotype 2,3
- Low viral load (less than 2 million copies/mL)
- No or minimal fibrosis
- Achieving EVR
- Female gender
- Short duration of disease
- Race (non-African American)

Variable

- Increasing physician experience
- PEG-IFN/RBV therapy (weight-based dosing; 24 weeks for Genotype 2,3; 48 weeks for Genotype 1)
- Adherence to therapy

treatment. Once treatment starts, however, one can use viral kinetic responses in the early stages of treatment to predict response. This is applicable to genotype 1 patients where early virological response (EVR) has been used to predict who is unlikely to have an SVR, a so-called stop rule. The advantages of EVR are that it reduces the morbidity and cost of treatment by stopping treatment in patients who are unlikely to respond [24]. To use viral kinetics, however, one needs to have reproducible and quantitative measurement of HCV RNA with no more than 0.5 $\log_{10}$ variability. Recent PCR tests are able to provide this accurate level of HCV RNA quantitation enabling physicians to use EVR for treatment decisions. The other important factor is to determine the primary goal of treatment, which is whether SVR alone is the endpoint of treatment or whether secondary benefits of therapy such as slowing disease progression or improving liver histology are applicable in the individual patient.

Early virological response is defined for treatment with both PEG-IFNs and RBV as either a 2 $\log_{10}$ unit reduction or loss of detectable HCV RNA at 12 weeks. When EVR does not occur, the chance of SVR being achieved by continuing the same treatment for 48 weeks is reduced to 1% to 3%, and an individualized decision can be made as to whether to stop treatment. For those patients who achieve EVR, there is an increased likelihood (65% to 70%) that they will have an SVR (Table 3).

Adherence to treatment

Another factor that has been reported to effect outcome is whether patients are able to tolerate therapy and are adherent to the planned treatment dose and duration. McHutchison looked at the effect of adherence in

Table 3
Effect of achieving EVR on hepatitis C virus treatment response

	Treatment response	
Early virological response (n)	SVR	NR
PEG-IFN alfa2b + RBV		
EVR ACHEIVED (388)	70%	30%
No EVR (124)	1%	99%
PEG-IFN alfa2a + RBV		
EVR ACHIEVED (390)	65%	35%
NO EVR (63)	3%	97%

patients treated with IFN/RBV and used the simple adherence parameters of whether patients were able to take 80% of their IFN, 80% of their RBV for 80% of the time, the 80/80/80 rule [25]. Approximately 30% of patients were unable to adhere to the treatment regimen, usually secondary to adverse effects of therapy. Inability to comply with therapy resulted in an overall loss of response that was more marked in genotype 1 patients, where SVR in the adherent group was 51% and fell to 34% in the patients who were dose-reduced or stopped therapy prematurely (Fig. 3). Factors that affect adherence include patient education and motivation, physician experience with adverse effect management, and positive reinforcement by physicians to the patient. The most successful centers treating HCV patients have incorporated these factors into overall management and often use physician extenders successfully in the role of primary caregivers to manage HCV adverse effects.

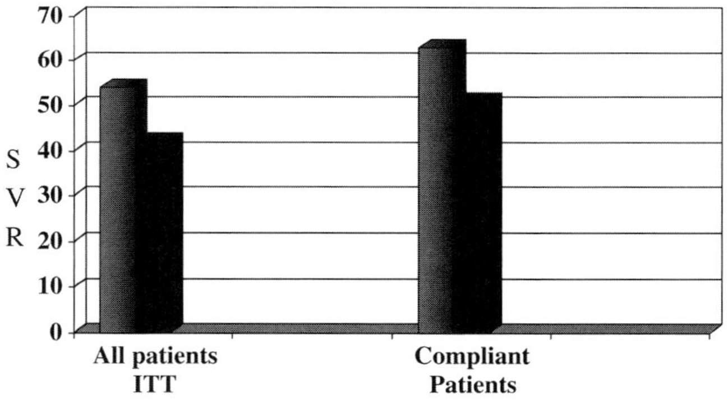

Fig. 3. Effect of adherence on SVR in patients treated with Peg-IFN alfa 2b 1.5 μg/kg and RBV 800 mg. The left panel shows the SVR for patients on intention-to-treat analysis (ITT), with the gray bars representing all patients and the black bars representing genotype 1 patients. Patients compliant to treatment by 80/80/80 rule had an increased SVR. All patients 54% to 63%, *p* 0.01; genotype 1 patients 42% to 51%, *P* greater than 0.03. (*Data from* McHutchison JG, Manns M, Patel K, Poynard T, Lindsay KL, Trepo C, et al. Adherence to combination therapy enhances sustained response in genotype-1-infected patients with chronic hepatitis C. Gastroenterology 2002;123(4):1061–9.)

Adverse effect management

The adverse effects of IFN and RBV are shown in Box 3, although a detailed discussion is beyond the scope of this article. One of the most frequent causes of dose reduction is the cytopenias associated with combination therapy. Thrombocytopenia with platelet counts of less than 50,000 usually is treated with dose reduction of IFN and is only seen in 1% to 4% of patients [26]. Neutropenia with neutrophils less than 750 per cc is seen in up to 20% of patients. No increased risk of bacterial infections has been reported with neutropenia, but dose reduction of IFN should be considered. Alternatively, use of growth factors such as granulocyte colony stimulating factor may be considered. Finally, anemia is common with combination therapy, with 50% of patients having a reduction of 3 g/dL in hemoglobin or a fall in hemoglobin to less than 12 g/dL [27]. Recent studies have shown that epoetin alfa at 40,000 U weekly can maintain RBV dose, improve hemoglobin by

Box 3. Common adverse effects of interferon/ribavirin therapy

Interferon

Bone marrow suppression
- Anemia
- Thrombocytopenia
- Neutropenia

Neuropsychiatric syndromes
- Depression
- Mood swings
- Anxiety/mania
- Neurocognitive dysfunction

Flulike syndrome
Nausea/gastrointestinal upset
Thyroid disease /thyroiditis
Alopecia
Neuropathy
Retinopathy
Injection site reactions

Ribavirin

Hemolytic anemia
Teratogenic
Dyspnea/cough
Rash/pruritis
Insomnia
Nausea/gastrointestinal upset

a mean of 2 g/dL, and improve quality of life in patients with IFN/RBV-induced anemia [28,29].

Interferon also is associated with several neuropsychiatric syndromes, including depression, mood swings, mania, anxiety, and neurocognitive dysfunction. Aggressive management of these side effects is necessary to maintain compliance to therapy.

In summary, remarkable improvements have been achieved in efficacy of treatment of naïve patients with HCV over the last decade, with SVR rates going from 10% to 50% with the current recommended PEG-IFN/RBV combination therapy. The success of therapy is dependent on many variables, and physicians who treat HCV should become very familiar with adverse effect management to achieve the results in clinical practice that have been demonstrated in the clinical trials to date.

Benefits and cost effectiveness of antiviral therapy

Follow-up of patients who have had an SVR for up to 10 years suggests that there is a persistent biochemical, virological, and histological remission in 95% of patients. This probably represents a true cure of HCV. It remains unknown if this translates into a reduction in the development of cirrhosis, liver failure, and HCC or translates into an improvement in survival. Economic and cost-effectiveness analyses have suggested that treatment of HCV has future cost savings comparable with many other accepted medical practices such as screening for colorectal cancer or hypertension and coronary artery bypass graft [30]. Finally, patients who have an SVR also have been shown to have significant improvements in health related quality of life, representing another strong argument for treating patients with HCV [31].

References

[1] Annual report of the US scientific registry for transplant recipients and the organ procurement and transplantation network-transplant data: 1988–1994. Richmond, VA: United Network for Organ Sharing and the Division of Organ Transplantation, Bureau of Health Resources Development.

[2] Alter MJ, Kruszon-Moran D, Nainan OV, McQuillan GM, Gao F, Moyer LA, et al. The prevalence of hepatitis C virus infection in the United States, 1988 through 1994. N Engl J Med 1999;341(8):556–62.

[3] Alter MJ. Epidemiology of hepatitis C. Hepatology 1997;26:62S–5.

[4] Recommendations for prevention and control of hepatitis C virus (HCV) infection and HCV-related chronic disease. Centers for Disease Control and Prevention. MMWR Morb Mortal Wkly Rep 1998;47(RR-19):1–39.

[5] Davis GL, Albright JE, Cook S, Rosenberg D. Projecting the future healthcare burden from hepatitis C in the United States. Hepatology 1998;28:390A.

[6] Marcellin P, Boyer N, Gervais A, Martinot M, Pouteau M, Castelnau C, et al. Long-term histologic improvement and loss of detectable intrahepatic HCV RNA in patients with

chronic hepatitis C and sustained response to interferon-alpha therapy. Ann Intern Med 1997;127(10):875–81.
[7] Marcellin P, Levy S, Erlinger S. Therapy of hepatitis C: patients with normal aminotransferase levels. Hepatology 1997;26:133S–6S.
[8] Sangiovanni A, Morales R, Spinzi G, Rumi M, Casiraghi A, Ceriani R, et al. Interferon alfa treatment of HCV RNA carriers with persistently normal transaminase levels: a pilot randomized controlled study. Hepatology 1998;27(3):853–6.
[9] Jacobson IM, Russo MW, Lebovics E, Esposito S, Tobias H, Klion F, et al. Interferon alfa-2b and ribavirin for patients with chronic hepatitis C and normal ALT: final results. Gastroenterology 2002;122:627.
[10] Sponseller C, Koehler KM, Hoffman JA, Strinko JM, Bacon BR. Use of interferon alpha-2b and ribavirin for treatment of patients with chronic hepatitis C with normal ALT levels. Hepatology 2002;36:579A.
[11] Hoofnagle JH, Mullen KD, Jones DB, Rustgi V, Di Bisceglie A, Peters M, et al. Treatment of chronic non-A, non-B hepatitis with recombinant human alpha interferon. A preliminary report. N Engl J Med 1986;315(25):1575–8.
[12] Davis GL, Balart LA, Schiff ER, Lindsay K, Bodenheimer HC Jr, Perrillo RP, et al. Treatment of chronic hepatitis C with recombinant interferon alfa. A multi-center randomized, controlled trial. Hepatitis Interventional Therapy Group. N Engl J Med 1989;321(22): 1501–6.
[13] McHutchison JG, Gordon SC, Schiff ER, Shiffman ML, Lee WM, Rustgi VK, et al. Interferon alfa-2b alone or in combination with ribavirin as initial treatment for chronic hepatitis C. Hepatitis Interventional Therapy Group. N Engl J Med 1998;339(21):1485–92.
[14] Di Bisceglie AM, Conjeevaram HS, Fried MW, Sallie R, Park Y, Yurdaydin C, et al. Ribavirin as therapy for chronic hepatitis C. A randomized, double-blind, placebo-controlled trial. Ann Intern Med 1995;123(12):897–903.
[15] Dusheiko G, Main J, Thomas H, Reichard O, Lee C, Dhillon A, et al. Ribavirin treatment for patients with chronic hepatitis C: results of a placebo-controlled study. J Hepatol 1996; 25(5):591–8.
[16] Bodenheimer HC Jr, Lindsay KL, Davis GL, Lewis JH, Thung SN, Seeff LB. Tolerance and efficacy of oral ribavirin treatment of chronic hepatitis C: a multi-center trial. Hepatology 1997;26(2):473–7.
[17] Poynard T, Marcellin P, Lee SS, Niederau C, Minuk GS, Ideo G, et al. Randomised trial of interferon alpha-2b plus ribavirin for 48 weeks or for 24 weeks versus interferon alpha-2b plus placebo for 48 weeks for treatment of chronic infection with hepatitis C virus. International Hepatitis Interventional Therapy Group (IHIT). Lancet 1998;352(9138):1426–32.
[18] Zeuzem S, Feinman SV, Rasenack J, Heathcote EJ, Lai MY, Gane E, et al. Peginterferon alfa-2a in patients with chronic hepatitis C. N Engl J Med 2000;343(23):1666–72.
[19] Lindsay KL, Trepo C, Heintges T, Shiffman ML, Gordon SC, Hoefs JC, et al. A randomized, double-blind trial comparing pegylated interferon alfa-2b to interferon alfa-2b as initial treatment for chronic hepatitis C. Hepatology 2001;34(2):395–403.
[20] Heathcote EJ, Shiffman ML, Cooksley WG, Dusheiko GM, Lee SS, Balart L, et al. Peginterferon alfa-2a in patients with chronic hepatitis C and cirrhosis. N Engl J Med 2000;343(23):1673–80.
[21] Manns MP, McHutchison JG, Gordon SC, Rustgi VK, Shiffman M, Reindollar R, et al. Peginterferon alfa-2b plus ribavirin compared with interferon alfa-2b plus ribavirin for initial treatment of chronic hepatitis C: a randomised trial. Lancet 2001;358(9286):958–65.
[22] Fried MW, Shiffman ML, Reddy KR, Smith C, Marinos G, Goncales FL Jr, et al. Peginterferon alfa-2a plus ribavirin for chronic hepatitis C virus infection. N Engl J Med 2002;347(13):975–82.
[23] Hadziyannis SJ, Cheinquer H, Morgan T, Diago M, Jensen DM, Sette H. Peginterferon alfa-2a (40kD)(PEGASYS) in combination with ribavirin (RBV): efficacy and safety results

from a phase III, randomized, double-blind multi-centre study examining effect of duration of treatment and RBV dose. J Hepatol 2002;36(Suppl 1):3.
[24] Davis GL, Wong JB, McHutchison JG, Manns MP, Harvey J, Albrecht J. Early virologic response to treatment with peginterferon alfa-2b plus ribavirin in patients with chronic hepatitis C. Hepatology 2003;38(3):645–52.
[25] McHutchison JG, Manns M, Patel K, Poynard T, Lindsay KL, Trepo C, et al. Adherence to combination therapy enhances sustained response in genotype-1-infected patients with chronic hepatitis C. Gastroenterology 2002;123(4):1061–9.
[26] Afdhal NH, Geahigan T. Supporting the patient with chronic hepatitis during treatment. In: Koff RS, Wu GY, editors. Clinical gastroenterology: diagnosis and therapeutics. Totowa (NJ): Humana Press. p. 211–32.
[27] Maddrey WC. Safety of combination interferon alfa-2b/ribavirin therapy in chronic hepatitis C-relapsed and treatment-naive patients. Semin Liver Dis 1999;19(Suppl 1): 67–75.
[28] Dieterich DT, Wasserman R, Brau N, Hassanein TI, Bini EJ, Sulkowski M. Once-weekly recombinant human erythropoietin (Epoetin Alfa) facilitates optimal ribavirin (RBV) dosing in hepatitis c virus (HCV) infected patients receiving interferon-alpha-2b (IFN)/RBV combination therapy. Gastroenterology 2001;120:340.
[29] Afdhal NH, Dieterich DT, Pockros PJ, Schiff ER, Shiffman M, Sulkowski M. Epoetin alfa treatment of anemic HCV-infected patients allows for maintenance of ribavirin dose, increases hemoglobin levels and improves quality of life vs. placebo: a randomized, double-blind, multi-center study. Gastroenterology 2003;124:714.
[30] Siebert U, Sroczynski G, Rossol S, Wasem J, Ravens-Sieberer U, Kurth BM, et al. Cost-effectiveness of peginterferon alpha-2b plus ribavirin versus interferon alpha-2b plus ribavirin for initial treatment of chronic hepatitis C. Gut 2003;52(3):425–32.
[31] Bonkovsky HL, Woolley JM. Reduction of health-related quality of life in chronic hepatitis C and improvement with interferon therapy. The Consensus Interferon Study Group. Hepatology 1999;29(1):264–70.

ELSEVIER
SAUNDERS

Infect Dis Clin N Am
20 (2006) 115–135

INFECTIOUS
DISEASE CLINICS
OF NORTH AMERICA

Approach to the Management of Patients with Chronic Hepatitis C Who Failed to Achieve Sustained Virologic Response

Amrita Sethi, MD, Mitchell L. Shiffman, MD*

Hepatology Section, Virginia Commonwealth University Medical Center, Box 980341, Richmond, VA 23298, USA

Therapy for chronic hepatitis C virus (HCV) infection has improved dramatically since interferon (IFN) was first introduced for treatment of non-A, non-B hepatitis over 15 years ago [1–3]. Historically, standard IFN monotherapy yielded a sustained virologic response (SVR) in less than 15% of patients. The addition of ribavirin (RBV) [4,5], and later the substitution of peginterferon (PEGIFN) for standard IFN [6–9], led to dramatic improvements in SVR rates, which can now be achieved in 45% to 50% of patients who have HCV genotype 1 and approximately 80% of patients who have genotypes 2 or 3 [10–12]. As each new improvement in HCV therapy has emerged, many patients who had failed to achieve SVR with previous, less effective therapy have been retreated. Recently, several large multicenter clinical trials have demonstrated the impact of retreating such patients with PEGIFN/RBV [13–16]. In the largest of these trials, 18% of patients who had a nonresponse (NR) after treatment with IFN or IFN/RBV achieved SVR after being retreated with PEGIFN/RBV. Certain subgroups, particularly those with previous relapse, HCV genotypes 2 and 3, without cirrhosis, or with low serum HCV RNA levels, faired better and seemed to be excellent candidates for retreatment (Table 1). In contrast, African Americans had a SVR of only 6%, and patients with multiple poor prognostic factors (HCV genotype 1, high serum HCV RNA levels, cirrhosis, and previous NR to IFN/RBV therapy) had poor SVR rates [13]. Given these findings, a thorough discussion regarding the pros and cons of retreatment should be

A version of this article originally appeared in the 8:2 issue of Clinics in Liver Disease.
Supported by NIH contract N01-DK-9-2322.
* Corresponding author.
E-mail address: mlshiffm@vcu.edu (M.L. Shiffman).

doi:10.1016/j.idc.2006.01.002

id.theclinics.com

Table 1
Response to retreatment with peginterferon and ribavirin in patients who failed to achieve sustained virologic response after treatment with interferon and ribavirin

	Sustained virologic response
Prior relapse to IFN/RBV[a]	40–50%
Prior nonresponse to IFN or IFN/RBV[b]	
Race	
Caucasian	20%
African American	6%
Genotype	
1	14%
non-1	60%
Serum HCV RNA level:	
<1.5 million IU/mL	31%
>1.5 million IU/mL	6%
Cirrhosis	
Yes	11%
No	23%

Abbreviations: IFN, interferon; RBV, ribavarin.
[a] *Data from* Ref. [14].
[b] *Data from* Refs. [13–15].

undertaken with each patient who failed to achieve SVR with IFN or IFN/RBV.

The majority of patients who have received therapy for chronic hepatitis C have been treated with PEGIFN/RBV as initial therapy or as retreatment after previous NR or relapse. No alternative with proven superiority is available for patients who have failed to achieve SVR after treatment with PEGIFN/RBV. Although the management of these patients represents a formidable challenge, several approaches are available that have the potential to yield SVR during retreatment or reduce the rate of disease progression. This article outlines an approach for managing patients who have failed to achieve SVR and reviews preliminary results of promising new therapies for these patients.

Identifying reasons for treatment failure

A number of factors may have contributed to the development of relapse or NR during previous therapy with PEGIFN and RBV. One possibility is that the patient was responding to treatment, had a marked decline in serum HCV RNA, and achieved early virologic response (EVR) or became HCV RNA undetectable (ie, the patient had a virologic response [VR], but this response was not recognized by the treating physician who subsequently discontinued therapy). Another possibility is that the physician significantly reduced the dosage of PEGIFN or RBV in the first several months of instituting treatment in response to the development of various side effects related to these medications. Finally, the patient may have been participating in behaviors that reduced the effectiveness of therapy. We refer to these three categories as "correctable factors"; the most important aspect of assessing a patient who has NR is to look for these factors because they can often be corrected before or during retreatment (Box 1). The successful correction of one or more of these factors has the potential to result in SVR during retreatment.

Failure to recognize virologic response

The use of testing for HCV RNA is essential to the diagnosis of HCV infection and to monitoring patients during therapy. Three basic methods are available to assess serum HCV RNA: polymerase chain reaction (PCR), branched chain DNA (b-DNA), and transmission mediated amplification (TMA). These assays, their limitations, and the proper manner by which virologic assays should be used to monitor HCV RNA during therapy were recently reviewed [17]. VR cannot be identified and patients cannot be appropriately monitored if the various HCV RNA response patterns that occur during therapy are not recognized. The definitions of VR were

Box 1. Factors that may increase the likelihood of sustained virologic response if corrected before or during retreatment

Failure to recognize virologic response

- HCV RNA not assessed during treatment
- HCV RNA not measured at the correct time during treatment
- Miscalculating the changes in HCV RNA from baseline during treatment
- Failure to account for natural variation in HCV RNA assays

Overly aggressive dose reduction

Significantly reducing the doses of PEGIFN and RBV during the first 24 weeks of treatment or stopping ribavirin before therapy is complete for the following reasons:

- Anemia
- Neutropenia
- Thrombocytopenia
- Severe flu-like symptoms
- Neuropsychiatric side effects
- Thyroid disease

Noncompliant behavior

- Continued alcohol use during treatment
- Continued illicit narcotic drug use during treatment
- Missed doses secondary to work or family/personal issues

developed during two National Institutes of Health (NIH) Consensus Development Conferences in 1997 and 2001 [18,19]; a graphic depiction of these definitions is provided in Fig. 1. Differentiating EVR, the null response, and partial VR is particularly important. EVR is defined as a 2-log (100-fold) or greater decline in the level of serum HCV RNA from the pretreatment baseline level or an undetectable HCV RNA 12 weeks after initiating IFN therapy. Virtually all patients with genotype 2 or 3 and 80% of treatment-naive patients with genotype 1 achieve EVR during PEGIFN/RBV therapy (Ferenci et al, submitted for publication, 2004) [20]. Approximately 65% of patients with an EVR achieve SVR. In contrast, SVR rarely, if ever, occurs in the absence of EVR.

VR occurs when a patient has an undetectable serum HCV RNA at any time during treatment. VR occurs in over 95% of patients who have genotypes 2 or 3 and in approximately 65% to 70% of patients who have genotype 1 by week 24 (Ferenci et al, submitted for publication, 2004). Only patients who achieve VR have the ability to develop SVR. However, approximately 10% of patients who have partial VR and detectable HCV RNA at treatment week 24 can become HCV RNA undetectable and achieve VR by week 48 if treatment is continued (Ferenci et al, submitted for publication, 2004). Although none of these patients will achieve SVR, the ability to become HCV RNA undetectable is potentially important for patients with chronic hepatitis C and advanced hepatic fibrosis or cirrhosis. The use of maintenance therapy for such patients is discussed below.

Null response is defined as the failure to achieve a 2-log decline in serum HCV RNA during the first 12 weeks of therapy. Patients with a null response rarely if ever have further decline in serum HCV RNA with continued therapy and are unlikely to respond during retreatment. Partial VR is defined by a 2-log or greater decline in serum HCV RNA from the pretreatment baseline value within 12 weeks but failure to become HCV RNA negative by treatment week 24. As opposed to the null response, patients who have a partial VR are excellent candidates for retreatment particularly if the

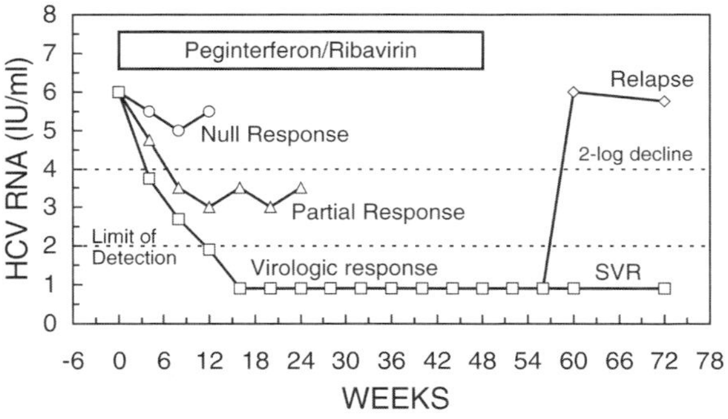

Fig. 1. Patterns of serum HCV RNA response during treatment.

factor or factors responsible for the failure to achieve VR can be identified and corrected.

In 1999, a universal standard for reporting serum HCV RNA was developed and implemented [17,21]. When reporting in international units, the most commonly used assays seem to be consistent with each other in their ability to measure serum HCV RNA [22,23]. However, like any other test, the values reported by any of these HCV RNA assays are subject to variability. The accuracy of the commercially available HCV RNA assays is reported to be ±0.5 log units [17,24,25], and this variation must be taken into account when assessing patients for EVR, as illustrated in Fig. 2. In this example, the patient had a baseline HCV RNA value of log 6 IU/mL (1 million IU/mL). Given the variability of the assay (±0.5 log units), the HCV RNA level may have been as high as log 6.5 IU/mL (3,162,278 IU/mL) or as low log 5.5 IU/mL (316,228 IU/mL). At 12 weeks of treatment, the HCV RNA level had declined by 2 log units to log 4 IU/mL (10,000 IU/mL), but, given the assay variability, the actual HCV RNA level could have been anywhere between log 4.5 IU/mL (31,623 IU/mL) and log 3.5 IU/mL (3162 IU/mL). Thus, EVR or a 2-log decline in the HCV RNA level from baseline could have occurred with a decline in HCV RNA of as little as 1 log unit, from log 5.5 IU/mL (316,000 IU/mL) to log 4.5 IU/mL (31,600 IU/ml), or as great as 3 log units, from log 6.5 IU/ml (3.16 million IU/ml) to log 3.5 IU/ml (31,600 IU/mL). Failure to recognize the variability in HCV RNA assays may lead the treating physician (or the patient's insurance carrier) to discontinue the patient's therapy at week 12 for falling just short of the 2-log decline in HCV RNA from the pretreatment baseline value (Fig. 3A). This scenario is one of the important correctable factors to look for when assessing patients who have NR.

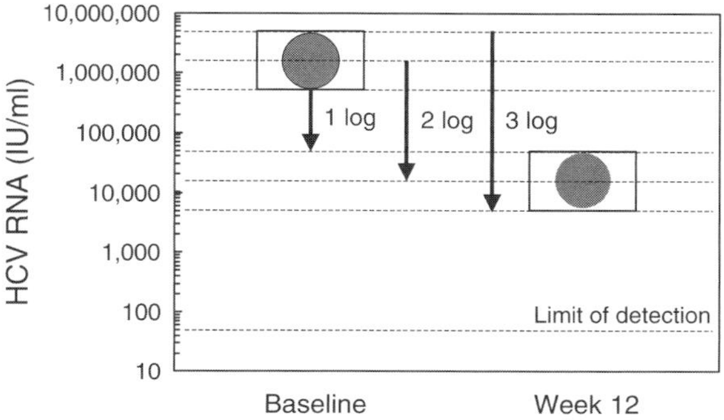

Fig. 2. Variations in serum HCV RNA results and how this can affect the ability to identify EVR. HCV RNA assays vary by ±0.5 log units, the range of which is highlighted by the shaded circles within the rectangular boxes. Because of this variability, a 2-log decline in the HCV RNA level may have occurred with only a 1-log decline and up to a 3-log unit decline in serum HCV RNA. This variability needs to be accounted for when assessing a patient for EVR during treatment.

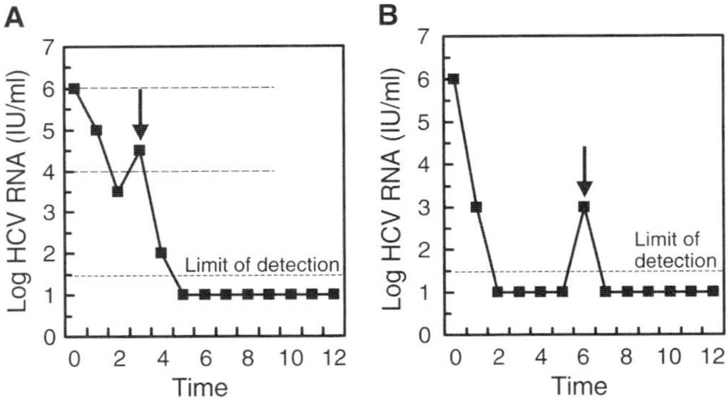

Fig. 3. Example of how more frequent testing of serum HCV RNA, particularly during the first 3 to 6 months of treatment, can improve recognition of EVR, VR, and the null response. (*A*) This patient was having a stepwise decline in HCV RNA at 1 and 2 months, but the value at 3 months was slightly higher and fell just short of a 2-log decline from baseline (*arrow*). By measuring serum HCV RNA monthly during the first 3 months of treatment, it was recognized that the patient already had a 2-log decline in serum HCV RNA at month 2 and that the elevation at 3 months could have represented assay variation. Treatment was continued, and the patient achieved VR by month 6. If only one HCV RNA value had been obtained at month 3 (*arrow*), treatment would have been discontinued, and the patient would have been labeled as an NR. (*B*) This patient had become HCV RNA undetectable by treatment month 2 but was HCV RNA positive at treatment month 6 (*arrow*). If HCV RNA had not been measured at monthly intervals, the patient might have been mischaracterized as an NR at month 6 and treatment discontinued. Because HCV RNA had been measured at monthly intervals, VR had been recognized. The positive HCV RNA value at month 6 was a discordant value, and treatment was continued.

Another important nuance of HCV RNA assays is the risk of false-positive and false-negative values. Recent studies have suggested that this may occur in up to 1% to 2% of samples assayed and is independent of the assay used [22,23]. Although false-negative results may be related to the lower limit of sensitivity in some assays [17,24], most discordant results seem to stem from sample processing errors that occur between the time blood samples are obtained, frozen, shipped to the reference laboratory, thawed, and pipetted into the amplification device used to measure HCV RNA. The reporting of a false-positive result when the sample is HCV RNA negative is another reason EVR or VR may not be recognized at weeks 12 and 24, respectively (Fig. 3B).

The recent recommendations to measure serum HCV RNA at baseline and week 12 in a patient with genotype 1 and to use only these values to determine EVR and whether treatment should be terminated or continued for 48 weeks may be insufficient to assess for variations in the HCV RNA assay or for the possibility of discordant results [26]. Examples of how more frequent monitoring of serum HCV RNA, particular during the first 3 to 6 months of therapy, can help the physician recognize EVR, VR, null response, and discordant results are provided in Fig. 3. The inability to recognize EVR or VR because HCV RNA was assessed too infrequently and treatment was discontinued prematurely is another potentially correctable factor when assessing patients who were thought to have NR.

Dose reduction and premature discontinuation of therapy

Approximately 20% to 30% of patients treated with IFN or PEGIFN and RBV develop adverse events sufficient to warrant dose reduction in one or both of these agents [10–12]. The major reasons to dose reduce PEGIFN include severe flu-like symptoms, neutropenia, thrombocytopenia, thyroid disorders, and psychiatric manifestations (eg, irritability and depression). The major reasons to dose reduce RBV include anemia, nausea, and rash. Aggressive management of these side effects has the potential to limit the number of patients who dose reduce or prematurely discontinue therapy [27].

Reducing the dose of PEGIFN or RBV seems to significantly impair the patient's ability to achieve EVR and SVR, particularly in patients with genotype 1 [13,28–30]. The degree by which the dose of PEGIFN or RBV can be reduced without adversely affecting SVR is controversial. In the first study to describe this association, SVR declined from 51% to 34% when PEGIFN or RBV was reduced to <80% of the starting dose at any time during the 48-week treatment course or if either of these agents was discontinued before the patient received 80% of the prescribed duration of therapy (ie, 36 weeks) [28]. This study assumed all dose reductions were equal and did not evaluate the impact of dose reducing PEGIFN or RBV independently or separate patients who dose reduced from those who prematurely discontinued treatment. The most critical time period for dose reduction seemed to be within the first 12 and 20 weeks of therapy. Patients who had a dose reduction before week 12 had a decline in SVR from 62% to 34%, whereas dose reduction after week 12 reduced SVR to only 51% [28]. In other studies, dose reducing PEGIFN or RBV after week 20 in patients who were HCV RNA undetectable had no impact on SVR as long as these agents were not stopped [13,29,30]. Preliminary data from a study of over 1100 patients with previous NR to IFN or IFN/RBV undergoing retreatment with PEGIFN/RBV demonstrated that the RBV dose could be reduced significantly during the first 20 weeks without affecting SVR as long as RBV was not discontinued and the PEGIFN dose was also not reduced [30].

Hematologic toxicities are the most common adverse events experienced by patients receiving PEGIFN and RBV, and anemia is the most common reason to dose reduce or discontinue RBV alone or both agents [10–12,27]. Anemia seems to be secondary to a combination of RBV-induced hemolysis and IFN-induced bone marrow suppression [31,32]. This most commonly occurs within the first 12 weeks of therapy, which is the most critical time for achieving EVR and is a time at which RBV use seems to be critical for enhancing SVR [13,27–30]. The mean decline in hemoglobin observed in patients treated with PEGIFN/RBV is 3 g, but declines of 4 g are routinely observed in over 20% of patients [33,34].

Identifying patients with relapse or NR who significantly reduced the dose or prematurely discontinued PEGIFN or RBV secondary to anemia is important when assessing patients with NR or relapse because this is a factor that could potentially be corrected or prevented during retreatment. Two studies have demonstrated that IFN/RBV-induced anemia can be corrected with epoetin alfa, which is also associated with a significant improvement in quality of life [35–37]. An example of how this agent can be used to prevent anemia and the need to dose reduce RBV in a patient with previous relapse is illustrated in Fig. 4. In this example, the patient developed severe anemia and had reduction in the doses of PEGIFN and RBV within the first 12 weeks. During retreatment, epoetin alfa was instituted early before the patient developed severe anemia, and the doses of PEGIFN and RBV were not reduced at any time during treatment, with the result that the patient achieved an SVR during retreatment.

Severe neutropenia can be corrected by using treatment with granulocyte colony-stimulating factor (GCSF), although no controlled trials of this agent have been performed in patients with chronic hepatitis C undergoing IFN therapy. Preliminary data have suggested that patients who have HCV who develop neutropenia are not at increased risk for bacterial or other infections [38]. As a result, the need for GCSF can probably be limited to

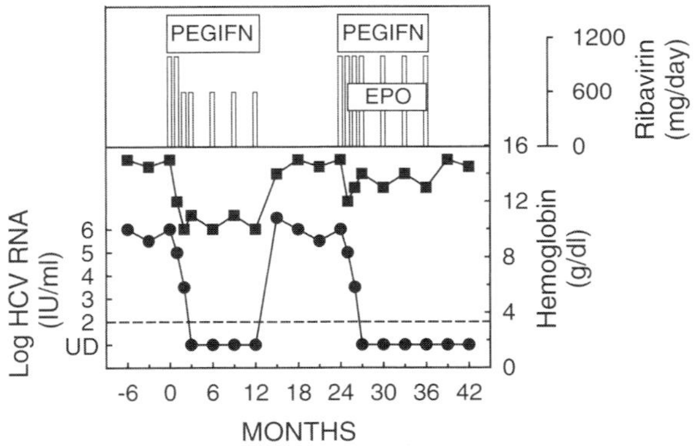

Fig. 4. Treatment of patient who had HCV with PEGIFN/RBV. During the first course of therapy, this patient developed severe anemia (hemoglobin <10 g/dL) and required discontinuation of RBV. The patient had already achieved EVR and was HCV RNA undetectable before RBV was discontinued and the PEGIFN dose reduced. As the hemoglobin rose, RBV was reinstituted, but at a lower dose (600 mg/d). The patient relapsed after 48 weeks of treatment. The patient was retreated with PEGIFN/RBV, and epoetin alfa (40,000 IU/week) was initiated as soon as the hemoglobin began to fall. No significant anemia developed. The patient remained on full-dose PEGIFN and RBV for 48 weeks and achieved SVR. UD: HCV RNA undetectable.

patients with a theoretical increased risk for bacterial infection. This includes patients with advanced cirrhosis awaiting liver transplantation, liver transplant recipients, and those with HIV coinfection. A reduction in the platelet count to values below 20,000/mL is rarely associated with spontaneous bleeding [39]. However, values this low are rarely observed during treatment with PEGIFN even in patients with cirrhosis. As a result, severe thrombocytopenia is an infrequent reason to dose reduce or discontinue treatment for chronic hepatitis C.

PEGINF may also need to be dose reduced or prematurely discontinued secondary to psychiatric side effects [10,11,27]. Psychiatric side effects severe enough to warrant intervention occur in about 20% to 33% of patients receiving PEGIFN/RBV, and these adverse events can frequently be treated with various antidepressant or antianxiety agents [40,41]. In contrast, some patients develop depression or irritability that is so severe and so rapid in its onset that dose reduction or discontinuation of treatment is necessary. Identifying such patients is important when assessing the reason for NR because this is a potentially correctable factor. Retreatment of these patients after their psychiatric disorder has been properly diagnosed and treated can be successful in achieving SVR.

Noncompliant patients

Many patients who begin IFN-based therapy for chronic HCV infection are not aware of the side effects of treatment or how to manage such side effects or regularly miss doses of PEGINF or RBV because of personal or work-related activities. Recent studies have demonstrated that the SVR rate may be up to 20% lower when patients are treated outside of organized clinical trials or by physicians who are relatively inexperienced at managing adverse events or who do not spend enough time educating patients regarding how to manage the side effects of PEGIFN and RBV [34]. Another type of noncompliance is consumption of large amounts of alcohol on a regular basis while receiving IFN therapy. Previous studies have demonstrated that alcohol use significantly reduces the SVR rate in patients being treated with IFN [42–44]. Similarly, ongoing or a recent history of injection drug use may affect the ability of patients to achieve SVR during treatment for chronic hepatitis C [45,46]. This NR seems to be secondary to a high rate of psychiatric side effects and noncompliance with the treatment regimen rather than to any specific antiviral effect of ongoing injection drug use. It is also possible that patients with ongoing drug abuse may become reinfected with a new strain of HCV during therapy.

Recognizing that noncompliance may have contributed to NR is important particularly if these factors can be addressed and corrected. Improving education and awareness regarding the side effects of PEGIFN and RBV, having a stronger commitment to therapy, or seeking care from a more experienced or attentive IFN provider may be useful for some patients. With proper counseling and support, some patients who consumed alcohol or used illicit drugs during previous therapy may achieve long-term abstinence. Noncompliance for any of these reasons is therefore an important correctable factor to address with patients who have failed to achieve SVR during previous therapy.

Therapies under investigation for the treatment of nonresponders

The list of new pharmaceutical agents being developed and evaluated as a possible treatment for patients with chronic HCV infection and NR to PEGIFN/RBV therapy was recently reviewed [47]. Some of the agents being evaluated in phase I and phase II clinical trials are listed in Table 2. By the time this issue of Infectious Disease Clinics is printed, it is likely that some of these agents will have failed clinical trials and no longer be under evaluation. It is equally likely that other agents will have completed preclinical development and will have entered the clinical trials arena as a potential treatment for patients with chronic HCV infection and previous NR or relapse. Numerous compounds in preclinical development are not listed in Table 2 because it is impossible to know which of these agents will enter

Table 2
Investigational agents for chronic hepatitis C nonresponders being investigated in clinical trials

Agent	Company	Description
CPG 10101	Coley	Stimulates production of many different endogenous IFNs Effect on serum HCV RNA unknown
NM283	Idenix	HCV protease inhibitor being evaluated as combination therapy with PEGIFN
1DN-I566	Idun	Caspase inhibitor reduces apoptosis Has no effect on serum HCV RNA level but seems to reduce serum ALT
ISIS 14803	ISIS	Oligonucleotide being evaluated as combination therapy with PEGIFN
Maximine	Maxim	Histamine analog being evaluated as combination therapy with PEGIFN
Thymosin alfa-1	Sciclone	Immune modulatory agent being evaluated as combination therapy with PEGIFN
Viramadine	Valaent	Ribavirin analog that does not cause hemolysis Being evaluated as combination therapy with PEGIFN
VX-950		HCV Ns3*4A protease inhibitor being evaluated as monotherapy Significant reduction in HCV RNA and serum ALT levels
SCH 503034		HCV protease inhibitor being evaluated in combination therapy with PEG-IFN. Seems to reduce HCV RNA
Albuferon		Genetically fused interferon alpha with serum human albumin Increased dosing interval of two to four weeks

Abbreviations: ALT, alanine aminotransferase; HCV, hepatitis C virus; IFN, interferon; IMPDH, inosine monophosphate dehydrogenase; PEGIFN, peginterferon; RBV, ribavirin.

clinical trials or be discarded during preclinical testing. Pharmaceutical companies, clinical research organizations, and governmental web sites can help patients and physicians to remain abreast of drug development and emerging clinical trials with new agents for patients with chronic hepatitis C.

Several agents available to physicians are being evaluated in clinical trials as a potential treatment for patients with chronic HCV infection and NR to previous PEGIFN/RBV therapy. Other trials are investigating the efficacy of higher doses of IFN or PEGIFN or a longer duration of therapy with these agents. Several of these strategies are discussed here because they may potentially be used by physicians for their patients with chronic hepatitis C. Only preliminary data are available regarding the use of these agents in this "off-label" manner. Discussing these approaches in this article does not advocate their use or suggest that they may be effective for treatment of patients who have HCV infection and NR to PEGIFN/RBV. Safety and efficacy will be determined when the results of these ongoing trials become available.

Protease inhibitors

Anti-viral therapy with first generation protease inhibitors has been undergoing evaluation for the past few years. Initially, significant results were seen with BILN 2061 used as monotherapy with 3 log reductions in HCV RNA. Studies were halted, however, after the development of cardiac toxicities in animal models [48]. The enthusiasm for this class of agents has been renewed with the development of three new drugs, NM283, VX-950, and SCH 503034. Each of these agents have been shown to significantly suppress HCV RNA when used either alone or in combination with PEGIFN [49–51]. Given prior experience with these agents, and the early phase of their trials, therapy with anti-HCV protease inhibitors should be approached with caution. Further studies of their use in combination therapy with interferon or triple therapy with interferon and ribavirin need to be evaluated.

Consensus interferon and ribavirin

Consensus interferon (CIFN) is a synthetic IFN product with an amino acid sequence that reflects all α-IFNs. CIFN has been shown to be effective in the retreatment of patients who failed to achieve SVR after 24 weeks of treatment with standard IFN monotherapy [52]. In that study, SVR was achieved in 58% of patients with previous relapse and in 13% with previous NR. High-dose daily CIFN using an "induction" approach has recently been evaluated for patients who have NR after treatment with PEGIFN/RBV in two small, single-center trials [53,54]. In one of these studies, CIFN was administered at doses of 27 or 18 μg daily for 4 weeks followed by 18 or 9 μg daily for 8 weeks, followed by 9 μg daily plus RBV (1000–1200 mg/d) for an additional 36 weeks. In the other study, CIFN was dosed at 15 μg/d plus RBV (1000–1200 mg/d) for 12 weeks followed by CIFN

15 μg TIW and RBV (1000–1200 mg/d) for 36 weeks. Preliminary data from these studies suggested that 37% to 42% of patients with previous PEGIFN/RVN could achieve SVR with these high-dose daily CIFN treatment regimens. One of these studies has suggested that this approach may be particularly helpful in African Americans [54], a group with a significantly lower SVR to PEGIFN/RBV therapy [55]. Based upon these single-center preliminary studies, a large, multicenter, clinical trial has been initiated in which CIFN (15 or 9 μg/d) plus RBV (1000–1200 mg/d) is being evaluated for the treatment of HCV patients with NR to previous PEGIFN/RBV therapy. Until this trial has been completed and this approach has been shown to have a positive impact, the use of high-dose daily CIFN along with RBV should be considered "off-label" and investigational.

Higher doses and longer duration of peginterferon and ribavirin

Another approach to the retreatment of patients who have NR to PEGIFN/RBV is to use these same agents but at a higher dose. In a preliminary study, patients with previous NR to IFN/RBV were retreated with 180, 270, or 360 μg of PEGIFNα-2a and RBV (1000–1200 mg/d). Although VR at the end of treatment was similar in all three groups, SVR increased stepwise from 21% to 46% in the highest PEGIFN dose group [56]. The increase in SVRs observed with higher doses of PEGIFN/RBV was therefore the result a marked reduction in relapse after discontinuation of this therapy. These data have led to the initiation of multicenter trials in which higher doses of PEGIFN and RBV are being used in patients who have NR to previous treatment with PEGIFN/RBV.

It has been hypothesized that patients who relapse after treatment with PEGIFN/RBV may have not been treated long enough to achieve long-lasting viral suppression. Preliminary results from a treatment trial in which patients were randomized to receive 48 or 72 weeks of therapy has demonstrated that relapse was reduced from 48% to 13% in patients treated for a longer period of time [57]. This study suggested that genotype 1 patients who relapsed after a standard course of PEGIFN/RBV may fare better if retreated for a longer period of time. The duration of retreatment and doses necessary to optimize SVR using this approach remains to be defined. In contrast, current data suggest that retreating patients with genotype 2 or 3 for a longer duration does not affect SVR because 24 and 48 weeks of therapy yield similar rates of SVR [12].

Peginterferon, ribavirin, and amantadine

Amantadine is an antiviral agent initially used for the treatment of influenza A [58]. Over the past several years, studies have investigated the possible role of amantadine for the treatment of chronic HCV infection. Amantadine has been used alone [59], with IFN [60], and as triple therapy with IFN and RBV [61,62] as initial therapy and for retreatment of patients with previous NR. Although most of these studies have yielded conflicting results, a recent meta-analysis has demonstrated that SVR might be about 5% to 7% higher in patients who received amantadine as part of triple therapy compared with IFN/RBV [63]. Preliminary reports evaluating amantadine, PEGIFN, and RBV triple therapy in patients with chronic HCV and previous NR remain inconclusive [64,65]. It is unclear what role amantadine will play in the management of patients who have failed to achieve SVR with PEGIFN/RBV.

Maintenance therapy

It is well established that patients who achieve SVR have an improvement in liver histology, a reduction in hepatic fibrosis [66–68], a reduced risk for developing hepatocellular carcinoma [69,70], and prolonged survival [70,71]. In contrast, it is doubtful that patients with NR achieve such benefit. Although it does seem that some nonresponders can achieve histologic improvement, this is probably limited to patients with partial VR and a marked decline in serum HCV RNA from the pretreatment baseline level [66,67,72]. Furthermore, the improvement in liver histology associated with partial VR seems to be limited to changes in hepatic inflammation. An overall improvement in liver fibrosis has not been convincingly demonstrated to occur in patients with NR after a single course of IFN [66,72]. Although one study implied that marked regression in fibrosis may occur in some patients with NR, this is unlikely because an equal percentage of patients in this study had fibrosis progression, over 60% of patients had no change in fibrosis, and the mean fibrosis scores from before and after treatment were not significantly different [68]. It is therefore, most likely that sampling variation accounted for the improvement in fibrosis reported to occur in a subset of patients who had NR.

Fibrosis progression in patients who have chronic HCV is mediated by hepatic inflammation [73,74]. As a result, it is possible that a reduction in hepatic inflammation may reduce the rate of fibrosis progression or allow fibrosis to resolve. This hypothesis forms the basis for the concept of maintenance therapy.

Maintenance therapy using interferon

Maintenance therapy using standard IFN was evaluated in a controlled trial of patients who achieved partial VR and a reduction in hepatic inflammation after an initial course of IFN therapy [72]. These patients were randomly assigned to continue IFN for an additional 2 years or to stop treatment and be followed as a control group. Patients who remained on IFN (3 MU tiw) therapy maintained the initial reduction in serum HCV RNA and improvement in hepatic inflammation observed after initial therapy. In contrast, serum HCV RNA and hepatic inflammation returned to the pretreatrnent baseline in patients randomized to stop therapy. Changes in mean fibrosis scores after 2.5 years in these two groups of patients were small and not statistically significant. Nevertheless, these findings were encouraging and led to the initiation of a several large, multicenter clinical trials to investigate the possibility that long-term maintenance therapy using PEGIFN could prevent fibrosis progression, reduce hepatic decompensation, lower the incidence of hepatocellular carcinoma, reduce the need for liver transplantation, and improve survival in patients who have HCV with NR and advanced fibrosis or cirrhosis. The HALT-C trial is the largest and most well publicized of these studies [75].

Preliminary results from another trial of maintenance PEGIFN (Co-Pilot) have recently been reported [76]. After 2 years of maintenance therapy (PEGIFNα-2b 0.5 μg/kg/wk), a significant reduction in the incidence of variceal hemorrhage was observed compared with patients treated with colchicine. No reduction in the incidence of liver failure, the development of hepatocellular carcinoma, the need for liver transplantation, or death was observed. This suggests that continuing PEGIFN as maintenance therapy may selectively reduce portal pressure but may not affect the natural progression of chronic hepatitis C in patients who have advanced fibrosis or cirrhosis.

Final results from the various clinical trials evaluating PEGIFN maintenance therapy will not be available for several years. Based upon available data, it is possible to consider maintenance therapy for patients with advanced fibrosis or stable cirrhosis who have relapsed after treatment with PEGIFN/RVN and who can tolerate the side effects of long-term treatment. Initiating PEGIFN at full dose and gradually tapering the dosage every 3 months to the lowest dose that maintains HCV RNA undetectable is a rational approach to patients with chronic HCV infection and advanced fibrosis or cirrhosis. In contrast, maintenance therapy should probably not be considered at this time in patients who have already developed complications of cirrhosis, in patients who do not achieve VR during treatment with PEGIFN and RBV, or in patients who do not remain HCV RNA undetectable with maintenance PEGIFN monotherapy. There are no data to suggest that patients who remain HCV RNA positive while on maintenance therapy achieve significant benefit from ongoing treatment.

Maintenance therapy using ribavirin

One study has evaluated the benefit of continuing RBV as maintenance therapy in patients who have HCV with NR [77]. Although RBV monotherapy does not reduce serum HCV RNA levels, serum alanine aminotransferase (ALT) declines significantly [78]. This implies that RBV may act as an anti-inflammatory agent to reduce hepatic inflammation and serve as a basis for the use of RBV as maintenance therapy. In this pilot trial, 38 patients who had NR to IFN/RBV were randomized to discontinue IFN and remain on RBV (1000–1200 mg/d) or placebo. After discontinuation of IFN, serum HCV RNA levels rose back to the pretreatment baseline levels in both groups. Although mean serum ALT levels also rose after discontinuation of IFN, patients who remained on RBV had a lower mean serum ALT levels compared with placebo-treated patients. After 48 weeks of RBV maintenance therapy, repeat liver biopsy demonstrated that 47% of patients had a significant decline in inflammation, whereas this was not observed in the placebo group. Although no significant improvement in fibrosis was observed with RBV maintenance therapy, the decline in hepatic inflammation suggests that this approach could be useful for the management of patients who have HCV with NR. It remains unknown which subgroup of patients who have NR could benefit from RBV maintenance therapy and if this decline in inflammation could be maintained without suppressing serum HCV RNA levels. As a result, the use of RBV as maintenance therapy should be considered un-proven at this time.

Modifying lifestyle factors associated with fibrosis progression

Many patients with chronic HCV infection and NR to PEGIFN/RBV have no, mild, or moderate fibrosis. Many of these patients are not at risk for developing fibrosis progression to cirrhosis for 5 to 15 years or longer [73,79,80]. It is estimated that 25% to 33% of patients who have chronic HCV infection will never develop fibrosis. It is therefore rational for many patients who have chronic HCV infection to be observed at periodic intervals until definitive improvements in therapy have been established. During this period, a focus on modifying lifestyle factors that seem to enhance fibrosis progression seems rational.

Several studies have demonstrated that patients who have HCV who consume alcohol on a regular basis have an increased rate of fibrosis progression to cirrhosis and a higher percentage of cirrhosis than patients who consume ethanol rarely or not at alt [42,43,79,81,82]. The minimum amount of alcohol that seems to be safe and not associated with an enhanced rate of fibrosis progression in HCV patients remains undefined. It is therefore prudent to counsel HCV patients not to consume alcohol except on rare occasions.

Another factor that seems to be associated with more rapid fibrosis progression to cirrhosis is hepatic steatosis secondary to nonalcoholic fatty liver disease (NAFLD). Several recent studies have suggested that patients who have chronic hepatitis C and NAFLD, or more importantly nonalcoholic steatohepatitis, have more fibrosis and a higher prevalence of cirrhosis than patients who have HCV infection without fatty liver [83,84]. NAFLD is strongly associated with obesity, insulin resistance, and hyperlipidemia and seems to be improved by weight loss, improved control of diabetes mellitus, and lowering of serum lipids [85,86], Such recommendations are strongly encouraged for patients with chronic HCV infection and coexistent NAFLD.

Patients who have chronic HCV infection should be vaccinated to prevent other forms of viral hepatitis [87,88]. A recent study has demonstrated that patients with chronic hepatitis C who acquire acute hepatitis A virus (HAV) are at increased risk for developing fulminant hepatic failure [89]. Although this same study did not find an increased risk of liver failure after acute infection with hepatitis B virus (HBV), patients coinfected with HCV and HBV seem to progress to cirrhosis at a faster rate [90]. Because exposure to HAV is sporadic and cannot be predicted, it is recommended that all patients with chronic HCV infection be vaccinated against HAV [87,88]. In contrast, the great majority of adults with acute hepatitis B acquired this infection by participating in some sort of risk behavior, most commonly sexual activity or illicit drug use. It is not always possible to predict which HCV patients might indulge in these risk behaviors. As a result, vaccination of patients with chronic HCV and NR against HAV and HBV seems prudent.

Summary

The combination of PEGIFN and RBV is the most effective therapy for patients with chronic hepatitis C. Although more than half of all patients are able to achieve SVR, a significant proportion of patients, particularly those with genotype 1, fail to have undetectable HCV RNA during treatment or relapse after completing therapy with return of detectable HCV RNA. An approach in the management of these patients is to identify factors that could have led to the NR or relapse and that could be corrected before or during a second course of therapy. Because fibrosis progression occurs slowly over decades for many patients with chronic hepatitis C, avoiding alcohol or other factors that could lead to fibrosis progression may be sufficient for the vast majority of patients. Other options that could be considered in patients who have more advanced disease include retreating with one of several new antiviral agents; retreating with higher doses of IFN or PEGIFN and RBV; or using IFN, PEGIFN, or RBV monotherapy long-term as maintenance therapy. The safety and efficacy of these approaches is being evaluated in numerous clinical trials.

References

[1] Hoofnagle JH, Mullen KD, Jones B, et al. Treatment of chronic non-A, non-B hepatitis with recombinant human alpha interferon. N Engl J Med 1986;315:1575–8.

[2] Thomson BJ, Doran M, Lever AML, et al. Alpha-interferon therapy for non-A, non-B hepatitis transmitted by gammaglobulin replacement therapy. Lancet 1987;1:539–41.

[3] Poynard T, Bedossa P, Chevallier M, et al. A comparison of three interferon alfa-2b regimens for the long-term treatment of chronic non-A, non-B hepatitis. N Engl J Med 1995; 332:1457–62.
[4] McHutchinson JG, Gordon S, Schiff ER, et al. Interferon alfa-2b alone or in combination with ribavirin as initial treatment for chronic hepatitis C. N Engl J Med 1998;339: 1485–92.
[5] Poynard T, Marcellin P, Lee SS, et al. Randomized trial of interferon α2b plus ribavirin for 48 weeks or for 24 weeks versus interferon α2b plus placebo for 48 weeks for treatment of chronic infection with hepatitis C virus. Lancet 1998;352:1426–32.
[6] Reddy KR, Wright TL, Pockros PJ, et al. Efficacy and safety of pegylated (40-KD) interferon α-2a compared with interferon α-2a in non-cirrhotic patients with chronic hepatitis C. Hepatology 2001;33:433–8.
[7] Zeuzem S, Feinman SV, Rasenack J, et al. Peginterferon-alfa-2a in patients with chronic hepatitis C. N Engl J Med 2000;343:1666–72.
[8] Heathcote EJ, Shiffman ML, Cooksley WG, et al. Peginterferon Alfa-2a in patients with chronic hepatitis C and cirrhosis. N Engl J Med 2000;343:1673–80.
[9] Lindsay KL, Trepo C, Heintges T, et al. A randomized, double-blind trial comparing peginterferon alfa-2b to interferon alfa-2b as initial treatment for chronic hepatitis C. Hepatology 2001;34:395–403.
[10] Manns MP, McHutchinson JG, Gordon SC, et al. Peginterferon-alfa-2b plus ribavirin compared with interferon alfa-2b plus ribavirin for initial treatment of chronic hepatitis C: a randomized trial. Lancet 2001;358:958–65.
[11] Fried MW, Shiffman ML, Reddy KR, et al. Combination of peginterferon alfa-2a (40 kd) plus ribavirin in patients with chronic hepatitis C vims infection. N Engl J Med 2002;347: 975–82.
[12] Hadziyannis SJ, Sette H Jr, Morgan TR, et al. Peginterferon-alfa 2a and ribavirin combination therapy in chronic hepatitis C: a randomized study of treatment duration and ribavirin dose. Ann Intern Med 2004;140:346–55.
[13] Shiffman ML, Di Bisceglie AM, Lindsay KL, et al. Peginterferon alfa-2a and ribavirin in patients with chronic hepatitis C who have failed prior treatment. Gastroenterology 2004;126: 1015–23.
[14] Jacobsen IM, Ahmed F, Russo MW, et al. Pegylated interferon alfa-2b plus ribavirin in patients with chronic hepatitis C: a trial in prior nonresponders to interferon monotherapy or combination therapy and in combination therapy relapsers: final results. Gastroenterology 2003;124(Suppl 1):A-714.
[15] Herrine SK, Brown R Jr, Esposito S, et al. Efficacy and safety of peginterferon alfa-2a combination therapies in patients who relapsed on rebetron therapy. Hepatology 2002;36(Suppl 1): 358A.
[16] Krawitt EL, Lidofsky SD, Ferrentino N, et al. Efficacy of peginterferon alfa-2b plus ribavirin in patients with chronic hepatitis C previously unresponsive to interferon-based therapy. Hepatology 2002;36(Suppl 1):359A.
[17] Ferreira-Gonzalez A, Shiffman ML. Use of diagnostic testing for managing hepatitis C virus infection. Semin Liver Dis 2004;24(Suppl 2):9–18.
[18] Lindsay KL. Therapy of hepatitis C: overview. Hepatology 1997;27(Suppl 1):71S–7S.
[19] Lindsay KL. Introduction to therapy of hepatitis C. Hepatology 2002;36(Suppl 1):S114–20.
[20] Davis GL, Wong JB, McHutchison JG, et al. Early virologic response to treatment with peginterferon alfa-2b plus ribavirin in patients with chronic hepatitis C. Hepatology 2003;38: 645–52.
[21] Saldanha J, Lelie N, Heath A. Establishment of the first international standard for nucleic acid amplification technology assays for HCV RNA. WHO collaborative study group. Vox Sang 1999;76:149–58.
[22] Shiffman ML, Ferreira-Gonzalez A, Reddy KR, et al. Comparison of three commercially available assays for HCV RNA using the international unit standard: implications for

management of patients with chronic hepatitis C virus infection in clinical practice. Am J Gastroenterol 2003;98:1159–66.
[23] Anderson JC, Simonetti J, Fisher DG, et al. Comparison of different HCV viral load and genotyping assays. J Clin Viral 2003;28:27–37.
[24] Nolte FS, Fried MW, Shiffman ML, et al. Prospective multicenter clinical evaluation of AMPLICOR and COBAS AMPLICOR hepatitis C virus tests. J Clin Microbiol 2001;39: 4005–12.
[25] Morishima C, Gretch DR. Clinical use of hepatitis C virus tests for diagnosis and monitoring during therapy. Clin Liver Dis 1999;3:717–40.
[26] Davis GL. Monitoring of viral levels during therapy of hepatitis C. Hepatology 2002; 36(Suppl 1):S145–51.
[27] Shiffman ML. Side effects of medical therapy for chronic hepatitis C. Ann Hepatol 2004;3: 5–10.
[28] McHutchison JG, Manns M, Patel K, et al. Adherence to combination therapy enhances sustained response in genotype-1-infected patients with chronic hepatitis C. Gastroenterology 2002;123:1061–9.
[29] Hadziyannis S, Cheinquer H, Morgan T, et al. Peginterferon alfa-2a in combination with ribavirin: efficacy and safety results from a phase III randomized, double-blind, multicenter trial examining effect of duration of treatment and ribavirin dose. J Hepatol 2002; 36(Supp 1):3.
[30] Shiffman ML, Morgan TR, Ghany MG, et al. The impact of peginterferon and ribavirin dosing on sustained virologic response in patients with chronic hepatitis C virus undergoing retreatment in the HALT-C trial. HALT-C trial group. Hepatology 2004;40(Suppl 1):314A.
[31] De Franceschi L, Fattovich G, Turrini F, et al. Hemolytic anemia induced by ribavirin therapy in patients with chronic hepatitis C virus infection: role of membrane oxidative damage. Hepatology 2000;31:997–1004.
[32] Shiffman ML, Hermann CM, Sterling RK, et al. A randomized, controlled trial to determine if continuing ribavirin as monotherapy in patients who responded to interferon/ribavirin combination therapy will enhance sustained virologic response. J Infect Dis 2001;184: 405–9.
[33] Maddrey WC. Safety of combination interferon alfa-2b/ribavirin therapy in chronic hepatitis C-relapsed and treatment-naive patients. Semin Liver Dis 1999;19(Suppl l):67–75.
[34] Nichols M, Kugelmas M. Reasons for discontinuation of treatment of chronic hepatitis C: an interim analysis of the Frontier trial. Gastroenterology 2003;124(Suppl 1):A703.
[35] Dieterich DT, Wasserman R, Brau N, et al. Once-weekly epoetin alfa improves anemia and facilitates maintenance of ribavirin dosing in hepatitis C virus-infected patients receiving ribavirin plus interferon alfa. Am J Gastroenterol 2003;98:2491–9.
[36] Afdhal NH, Dieterich DT, Pockros PJ, et al. Correction of anemia with epoetin alfa maintains ribavirin dose in HCV-infected patients: a prospective, double-blind study. Gastroenterology 2004;126:1302–11.
[37] Pockros PJ, Shiffman ML, Schiff ER, et al. Epoetin alfa improves quality of life in anemic HCV-infected patients receiving combination therapy. Hepatology 2004;40:1450–8.
[38] Ahmed F, Jacobson IM, Brown RS Jr, et al. Neutropenia and infections in the WIN-R trial. Gastroenterology 2003;124(Suppl 1).
[39] Boks AL, Brommer EJ, Schalm SW, et al. Hemostasis and fibrinolysis in severe liver failure and their relation to hemorrhage. Hepatology 1986;6:79–86.
[40] Hauser P. Neuropsychiatric side effects of HCV therapy and their treatment focus on IFN alpha-induced depression. Gastroenterol Clin North Am 2004;33(Suppl 1):S35–50.
[41] Maddock C, Baita A, Orru MG, et al. Psychopharmacologic treatment of depression, anxiety, irritability and insomnia in patients receiving interferon-alpha: a prospective case series and a discussion of biologic mechanisms. J Psychopharmacol 2004;18:41–6.
[42] Schiff ER, Ozden N. Hepatitis C and alcohol. Alcohol Res Health 2003;27:232–9.
[43] Peters MG, Terrault NA. Alcohol use and hepatitis C. Hepatology 2002;36:S220–5.

[44] Loguercio C, Di Pierro M, Di Marino MP, et al. Drinking habits of subjects with hepatitis C virus-related chronic liver disease: prevalence and effect on clinical, virological and pathological aspects. Alcohol 2000;35:296–301.
[45] Edlin BR. Prevention and treatment of hepatitis C in injection drug users. Hepatology 2002; 36(Suppl 1):S210–9.
[46] Sylvestre DL, Clements BJ. The impact of negative prognostic factors on hepatitis C treatment outcomes in recovering injection drug users. Hepatology 2002;36:223A.
[47] McHutchison JG, Patel K. Future therapy of hepatitis C. Hepatology 2002;36:S245–52.
[48] Hinrichsen H, Benhamou Y, Wedemeyer H, et al. Short-term antiviral efficacy of BILN 2061, a hepatitis C virus serine protease inhibitor, in hepatitis C genotype 1 patients. Gastroenterology 2004;127:1347–55.
[49] O'Brien C, Godofsky E, Rodriquez-Torres M, et al. Randomized trial of valopicitabine (NM283) alone or with peg-interferon vs. retreatment with peg-interferon plus ribavirin in hepatitis C patients with previous non-response PEGIFN/RBV: first interim results [abstract #95]. Hepatology 2005;42:234A.
[50] Reesink HW, Zeuzem S, Weegink CJ, et al. Final results of a phase 1b, multiple dose study of VX-950, a hepatitis C virus protease inhibitor [abstract #96]. Hepatology 2005;42:234A–5A.
[51] Zeuzem S, Sarrazin C, Wagner F, et al. Combination therapy with the HCV protease inhibitor, SCH 503034, plus peg-intron in hepatitis C genotype 1 peg-intron non-responders: Phase 1b results [abstract #201]. Hepatology 2005;42:276A.
[52] Heathcote EJ, Keeffe EB, Lee SS, et al. Re-treatment of chronic hepatitis C with consensus interferon. Hepatology 1998;27:1136–43.
[53] Kaiser S, Hass H, Gregor M. Successful retreatment of peginterferon nonresponders with chronic hepatitis C with high dose consensus interferon induction therapy. Gastroenterology 2003;124(Suppl 1):A700.
[54] Leevy C II, Chamers C, Blatt L. Comparison of African American and non-African American patient end of treatment response for PEGIFN alpha-2a and weight based ribavirin nonresponders retreated with IFN alfacon-1 and weight based ribavirin. Hepatology 2004;40(Suppl 1):240A.
[55] Muir AJ, Bornstein JD, Killenberg PG. Peginterferon alfa-2b and ribavirin for the treatment of chronic hepatitis C in blacks and non-hispanic whites. N Engl J Med 2004;350: 2265–71.
[56] Diago M, Crespo J, Oliveira A, et al. Peginterferon alfa-2a and ribavirin in patients infected with HCV genotype 1 who failed to respond to interferon and ribavirin: final results of the Spanish high dose induction pilot trial. Hepatology 2004;40(Suppl 1):389A.
[57] Sanchez-Tapias JM, Diago M, Escartin P, et al. Hepatology 2004;40(Suppl 1):218A.
[58] Younossi ZM, Perrillo RP. The roles of amantadine, rimantadine, ursodeoxycholic acid and NSAIDs, alone or in combination with alfa interferons in the treatment of chronic hepatitis C. Semin Liver Dis 1999;19:95–102.
[59] Smith JP. Treatment of chronic hepatitis C with amantadine. Dig Dis Sci 1997;42:1681–7.
[60] Helbling B, Stamenic I, Viani F, et al. Interferon and amantadine in naive chronic hepatitis C: a double-blind, randomized, placebo-controlled trial. Hepatology 2002;35:447–54.
[61] Teuber G, Pascu M, Berg T, et al. Randomized, controlled trial with IFN-alpha combined with ribavirin with and without amantadine sulphate in non-responders with chronic hepatitis C. JHepatol 2003;39:606–13.
[62] Thuluvath PJ, Maheshwari A, Mehdi J, et al. Randomized, double blind, placebo controlled trial of interferon, ribavirin, and amantadine versus interferon, ribavirin, and placebo in treatment naive patients with chronic hepatitis C. Gut 2004;53:130–5.
[63] Mangia A, Leandro G, Helbling B, et al. Combination therapy with amantadine and interferon in naive patients with chronic hepatitis C: meta-analysis of individual patient data from six clinical trials. J Hepatol 2004;40:478–83.
[64] Fargion S, Borzio M, Predabissi O, et al. End of treatment and sustained response to peginterferon alfa-2a plus ribavirin and amantadine and to induction therapy with interferon

alfa-2a plus ribavirin and amantadine in interferon/ribavirin nonresponders with chronic hepatitis C. Hepatology 2003;38(Suppl 1):733A.
[65] Cantu NS, Davis M, Afdahl N, et al. Triple therapy compared to standard pegylated interferon alfa-2b and weight based ribavirin for previous nonresponders and relapsers with chronic hepatitis C. Hepatology 2003;38(Suppl 1):742A.
[66] Shiffman ML, Hermann CM, Thompson EB, et al. Relationship between biochemical, virologic and histologic response during interferon treatment of chronic hepatitis C. Hepatology 1997;26:780–5.
[67] Shiffman ML. Histologic improvement in response to interferon therapy in chronic hepatitis C. Viral Hepatitis Rev 1999;5:27–43.
[68] Poynard T, McHutchison J, Manns M, et al. Impact of pegylated interferon alfa-2b and ribavirin on liver fibrosis in patients with chronic hepatitis C. Gastroenterology 2002;122: 1303–13.
[69] Imai Y, Kawata S, Tamura S, et al. Relation of interferon therapy and hepatocellular carcinoma in patients with chronic hepatitis C. Ann Intern Med 1998;129:94–9.
[70] Yoshida H, Arakawa Y, Sata M, et al. Interferon therapy prolonged life expectancy among chronic hepatitis C patients. Gastroenterology 2002;123:483–91.
[71] Fattovich G, Giustina G, Degos F, et al. Effectiveness of interferon alfa on incidence of hepatocellular carcinoma and decompensation in cirrhosis type C. European concerted action on viral hepatitis. J Hepatol 1977;27:201–5.
[72] Shiffman ML, Hofmann CM, Contos MJ, et al. A randomized, controlled trial of maintenance interferon for treatment of chronic hepatitis C non-responders. Gastroenterology 1999;117:1164–72.
[73] Yano M, Kumada H, Kage M, et al. The long term pathological evolution of chronic hepatitis C. Hepatology 1996;23:1334–40.
[74] Ghany MG, Kleiner DE, Alter H, et al. Progression of fibrosis in chronic hepatitis C. Gastroenterology 2003;124:97–104.
[75] Lee WM, Dienstag JL, Lindsay KL, et al. Evolution of the HALT-C trial: pegylated interferon as maintenance therapy for chronic hepatitis C in previous interferon nonresponders. Control Clin Trials 2004;25:472–92.
[76] Afdhal N, Freilich B, Levine R, et al. Colchicine versus Peg-Intron long term (CoPilot) trial: interm analysis of clinical outcomes at year 2. Hepatology 2004;40(Suppl 1):239A.
[77] Hoofnagle JH, Ghany MG, Kleiner DE, et al. Maintenance therapy with ribavirin in patients with chronic hepatitis C who fail to respond to combination therapy with interferon alfa and ribavirin. Hepatology 2003;38:66–74.
[78] Di Bisceglie AM, Conjeevaram HS, Fried MW, et al. Ribavirin as therapy for chronic hepatitis C: a randomized, double-blind, placebo-controlled trial. Ann Intern Med 1995;123: 897–903.
[79] Poynard T, Bedossa P, Opolon P. Natural history of liver fibrosis progression in patients with chronic hepatitis C. The OBSVIRC, METAVIR, CLINVIR and DOSVIRC groups. Lancet 1997;349:825–32.
[80] Afdhal NH. The natural history of hepatitis C. Semin Liver Dis 2004;24(Suppl 2):3–8.
[81] Safdar K, Schiff ER. Alcohol and hepatitis C. Semin Liver Dis 2004;24:305–15.
[82] Wiley TE, McCarthy M, Breidi L, et al. Impact of alcohol on the histological and clinical progression of hepatitis C infection. Hepatology 1998;28:805–9.
[83] Ramesh S, Sanyal AJ. Hepatitis C and nonalcoholic fatty liver disease. Semin Liver Dis 2004; 24:399–413.
[84] Younossi ZM, McCullough AJ, Ong JP, et al. Obesity and non-alcoholic fatty liver disease in chronic hepatitis C. J Clin Gastroenterol 2004;38:705–9.
[85] Haynes P, Liangpunsakul S, Chalasani N. Nonalcoholic fatty liver disease in individuals with severe obesity. Clin Liver Dis 2004;8:535–47.
[86] Lonardo A, Adinolfi LE, Loria P, et al. Steatosis and hepatitis C virus: mechanisms and significance for hepatic and extrahepatic disease. Gastroenterol 2004;126:586–97.

[87] Reiss G, Keeffe EB. Review article: hepatitis vaccination in patients with chronic liver disease. Aliment Pharmacol Ther 2004;19:715–27.
[88] Strader DB, Wright T, Thomas DL, et al. Diagnosis, management, and treatment of hepatitis C. Hepatology 2004;39:1147–71.
[89] Vento S, Garofano T, Renzini C, et al. Fulminant hepatitis associated with hepatitis A virus superinfection in patients with chronic hepatitis C. N Engl J Med 1998;338:286–90.
[90] Sterling RK, Sulkowski MS. Hepatitis C virus in the setting of HIV or hepatitis B virus coinfection. Semin Liver Dis 2004;24(Suppl 2):61–8.

ELSEVIER
SAUNDERS

Infect Dis Clin N Am
20 (2006) 137–153

INFECTIOUS
DISEASE CLINICS
OF NORTH AMERICA

Treatment of Relapsers after Combination Therapy for Chronic Hepatitis C

Furqaan Ahmed, MD, Ira M. Jacobson, MD*

Division of Hepatology and Gastroenterology, Weill Medical College of Cornell University, 450 East 69th Street, New York, NY 10021, USA

The treatment for chronic hepatitis C (CHC) has evolved over the last decade from standard interferon (IFN) monotherapy to combination therapy with standard IFN and ribavirin (RBV) and more recently, pegylated (PEG) IFN and RBV combination therapy. As each successive regimen has led to improved sustained virologic response (SVR) rates, the issue of retreating those patients who did not achieve a sustained response with previous therapy arises. A relapse after therapy is defined as viral clearance with a negative hepatitis C virus (HCV) RNA by polymerase chain reaction (PCR) during therapy and reappearance of the virus after treatment is discontinued. This article focuses on the treatment of patients who have relapsed after being treated with IFN or a combination of IFN and RBV. Relapse to PEG IFN and RBV will also be discussed.

Rates of relapse

Studies with standard IFN monotherapy at 3 million units three times weekly have demonstrated SVR rates after 24 and 48 weeks of therapy to be 6% and 13% to 19%, respectively [1,2]. RBV was approved by the US Food and Drug Administration (FDA) for the treatment of CHC in combination with IFN in 1998. RBV's mechanism of action, a nucleoside analog, has still not been elucidated firmly. Postulated mechanisms include

Dr. Jacobson is a consultant and has received research support from Schering-Plough.

A version of this article originally appeared in the 33:3 issue of Gastroenterology Clinics of North America.

* Corresponding author.

E-mail address: imj2001@med.cornell.edu (I.M. Jacobson).

doi:10.1016/j.idc.2006.01.010 *id.theclinics.com*

inhibition of host inosine monophosphate dehydrogenase, enhancement of host T-cell mediated immunity against HCV, direct HCV inhibition, and increased HCV RNA mutagenesis leading to error catastrophe [3,4]. Recent viral kinetic studies favor one or more antiviral rather than immunomodulatory mechanisms [5]. Although ineffective in the treatment of CHC as monotherapy [6–8], when administered with IFN, RBV increases SVR rates by increasing response rates and, even more notably, by decreasing the rate of post-treatment relapse in patients who become HCV RNA-negative on therapy. The combination of standard IFN and RBV therapy for 24 weeks in naïve patients results in end-of-treatment viral clearance rates of 53% to 57% and SVR rates of 31% to 35% [1,2]. Combination therapy for 48 weeks results in end-of-treatment response rates of 50% to 52% and SVR rates of 38% to 43% [1,2]. Prolongation of combination standard interferon and ribavirin therapy to 72 weeks does not result in significantly higher SVR rates (43%) than that achieved with 48 weeks of therapy [9]. The incremental efficacy of 48 weeks or 72 weeks versus 24 weeks of therapy appears to be limited to patients with HCV genotype 1 infection.

Pegylated IFNs, developed by the covalent attachment of a polyethylene glycol molecule to standard IFN, have a longer half-life and increased therapeutic efficacy. PEG IFN alfa-2b and alfa-2a have been approved by the FDA for the treatment of CHC in combination with RBV, and this therapy represents the current standard of care for CHC. Two landmark studies evaluated the efficacy of PEG IFN alfa-2a and alfa-2b and RBV treatment. PEG IFN alfa-2b at 1.5 μg/kg per week and RBV (800 mg per day) in naïve patients led to end-of-treatment response rates of 65% and SVR rates of 54% [10]. PEG IFN alfa-2a at 180 μg per week and RBV (1000 to 1200 mg) resulted in end-of-treatment response rates of 69% and SVR rates of 56% [11]. Even with these newer treatment regimens that result in higher SVR rates, a significant number of patients relapse when therapy is stopped. The relapse rates are lower than they were with older forms of therapy, however.

Clearance of HCV viremia with antiviral therapy followed by relapse is associated with improvements in liver histology and reductions in the development of liver complications that are in-between those seen in patients who achieve SVR and those who are nonresponders to anitiviral therapy [12,13].

Mechanisms of relapse

The precise reason for HCV relapse is likely multifactorial and may result from host-, viral-, and treatment-related factors. Differences in HCV genotypes influence response to therapy. Genotype 1 is more resistant to therapy than genotypes 2 and 3, and patients with genotype 1 who achieve a response on treatment have slightly higher rates of relapse after discontinuation of therapy, even with PEG IFN alfa-2b and RBV [14]. Similarly, patients with advanced fibrosis have higher rates of relapse, particularly with IFN monotherapy [14].

The host immune response plays a pivotal role in determining the ultimate outcome of therapy. Also, factors including age, ethnicity, and the degree of liver fibrosis influence treatment outcome. The development of anti-IFN neutralizing antibodies may play a role for some patients who have viral breakthrough during therapy [15,16]. The importance of these antibodies in patients who relapse after therapy is discontinued is doubtful, however. Other host factors not yet identified also may predispose some patients to fail to clear the virus completely from the liver.

A two-phase model of viral clearance after initiation of IFN therapy has been described [17]. The first phase, consisting of a rapid decline in viremia, results from IFN-induced inhibition of HCV virion production. The second and more gradual decline in viremia represents HCV-infected cell death (Fig. 1). This model suggests that relapsers are patients who have not cleared all virus-infected hepatocytes at the time their treatment is stopped. This hypothesis is supported by studies using transcription mediated amplification, a recently developed sensitive viral assay (>5 IU/mL), which detected low levels of HCV viremia in retrospectively analyzed stored serum samples of up to 36% of patients who were classified as end-of-treatment responders by conventional PCR tests but subsequently relapsed [18].

Because of the practical obstacles to serial liver biopsy and the challenges in quantifying intrahepatic virus, it is unknown whether there is progressive attrition of infected cells or whether, in some patients, the process achieves a plateau beyond which further clearance does not occur. Similarly, it is unknown whether the mechanism of intrahepatic viral persistence represents some form of latency or simply very low viral replication undetectable in serum. As a flavivirus, however, it is presumed that HCV is not capable of genomic integration, as is the case with HIV and hepatitis B virus (HBV).

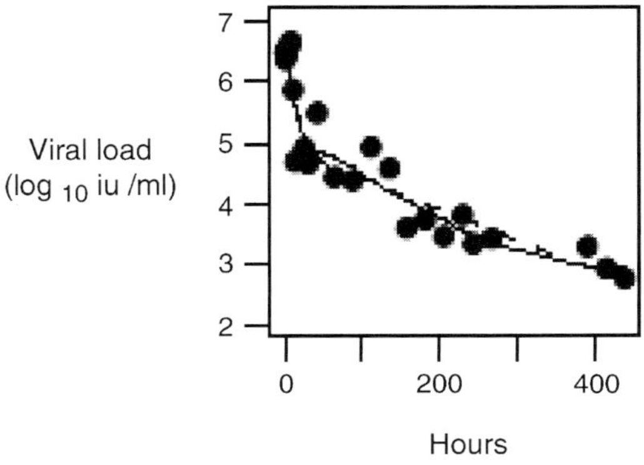

Fig. 1. Two phase model of viral clearance with interferon therapy. The first, steeper phase is thought to be related to inhibition of viral production, while the second, more gradual phase, represents clearance of infected hepatocytes. (*Courtesy of* Gerond Lake-Bakaar, MD.)

Retreatment of interferon monotherapy relapsers with interferon alone or with combination interferon and ribavirin therapy

Several studies have evaluated retreatment of patients who relapsed after IFN monotherapy. Retreating patients who relapsed after a course of standard IFN at 3 million units three times weekly for 24 weeks with the same regimen has not been shown to be efficacious, with SVR rates of only 0% to 5% [19–21], although a few studies have reported higher SVR rates [22,23]. Retreatment with standard IFN at 3 million units three times weekly but for a longer duration results in higher SVR rates. Forty-eight weeks of therapy has led to SVR rates of 29% to 36% [22,23]. Treatment for 96 weeks has resulted in SVR rates of 68% [22].

Other investigators have retreated relapsers with higher doses of standard IFN for 24 weeks. IFN doses of 4.5 to 5 million units three times weekly for 24 weeks were reported to induce an SVR in 35% to 38% of monotherapy relapsers [19,24]. Studies using even higher doses of IFN, however, have reported lower SVR rates. One study using 6 million units three times weekly resulted in an SVR in 5% of patients [25], and a dose of 10 million units resulted in an SVR of 18.5% [23]. Cavaletto et al treated 25 patients with an 8-week induction phase of 6 million units three times weekly, followed by 3 million units for 24 weeks and reported an SVR rate of 16% [26]. It is unclear why the highest doses of IFN therapy resulted in lower SVR rates.

Chow et al combined both approaches to the retreatment of patients who have relapsed to prior therapy using both a higher dose of IFN and a longer duration of therapy [19]. They treated 11 patients with 5 million units of IFN three times weekly for 48 weeks and reported an SVR rate of 27%, which was lower than the SVR rate in patients treated with 5 million units of IFN for 24 weeks (35%).

Retreatment of IFN monotherapy relapsers with combination standard IFN and RBV results in higher SVR rates than retreatment with IFN alone. Davis et al retreated patients with IFN (3 million units three times weekly) and RBV for 24 weeks and reported an SVR rate of 49%, markedly higher than SVR rates in patients who were retreated with IFN monotherapy for 24 weeks (5%) [20]. Similar SVR rates of 25% to 40% have been reported in most studies retreating IFN monotherapy relapsers with IFN and RBV combination therapy [25,27–29]. One study reported an SVR rate of 75% in 20 patients treated with this regimen [30]. Similar or slightly higher rates of SVR (29% to 49%) have been reported when patients are treated with higher doses of IFN (5 to 6 million units three times weekly) and RBV for 24 weeks [24,29,31].

Reported SVR rates after 48 weeks of IFN at 3 million units three times weekly and RBV range from 40% to 67% [27,29,32]. Forty-eight weeks of high-dose (5 to 6 million units) IFN and RBV therapy resulted in SVR rates of 47% to 72% [29,31,32]. Cavaletto treated 25 patients with an 8-week induction phase of 6 million units three times weekly, followed by 3 million units of standard IFN in addition to RBV (1000 to 1200 mg per day) for 24 weeks and reported an SVR rate of 44% [26]. In another study, biochemical relapsers were retreated with a 24 week course of high dose IFN (6 million units three times weekly) followed by 3 million units three times weekly for 24 weeks with or without ribavirin (for 24 or 48 weeks) [33]. SVR rates in patients with low HCV viral load (less than 2 million copies/mL, n = 89) were significantly greater in patients who also received RBV (600 mg daily for the first 24 weeks) compared with IFN monotherapy alone (59.6% versus 37.7%, $P < 0.05$). In patients with a high viral load (greater than 2 million copies/mL, n = 208), SVR rates were 44.7% and 51.4% in patients treated with RBV (600 mg daily) for 24 weeks and 48 weeks, respectively. Genotype non-1, Knodell score of less than 6 on liver biopsy, and ALT level greater than three times the upper limit of normal were associated with a greater likelihood of achieving an SVR.

Shiffman et al randomized patients with an end-of-treatment virologic response after 24 weeks of IFN and RBV to either discontinue therapy or continue RBV monotherapy for 24 additional weeks [30]. Of the 46 patients with an end-of-treatment response, SVR rates were 75% in the group that discontinued therapy and 50% in the group treated with RBV monotherapy, indicating that continuing RBV monotherapy after achieving a virologic response does not increase the likelihood of an SVR. Krawitt et al treated 17 IFN monotherapy relapsers with PEG IFN alfa-2b (100 to 150 µg per week) and RBV (1000 mg daily); 53% had an SVR [34].

In conclusion, retreatment with the same treatment regimen for the same duration of therapy has not been shown to result in significant SVR rates in patients who have relapsed after a previous course of therapy previously. In contrast, higher doses, and, more importantly, longer duration of therapy lead to significant SVR rates in these groups. It is also important to remember that when IFN monotherapy relapsers are treated with standard IFN and RBV or PEG IFN and RBV therapy, much of the increase in SVR rates undoubtedly reflects the incremental increase in SVR associated with combination therapy regardless of whether treatment duration is extended.

Treatment of patients who have relapsed after interferon and ribavirin combination therapy

Data on the retreatment of patients who have relapsed after combination therapy with standard IFN and RBV are more limited. There are no data on retreating these patients with regimens of standard IFN and RBV. In a few studies mostly reported only in abstract form, combination relapsers have been retreated with PEG IFN and RBV (Table 1).

Jacobson et al randomized patients who had relapsed after IFN and RBV therapy to receive 48 weeks of either PEG IFN alfa-2b 1.0 µg/kg per week and RBV 1000 to 1200 mg per day or PEG IFN alfa-2b 1.5 µg/kg per week and RBV 800 mg per day [35]. Twenty five patients received the higher dose

Table 1
Combination peginterferon and ribavirin for relapses to standard interferon and ribavirin

Author	Patient number	Treatment regimen	Overall end of treatment response (%)	Overall SVR (%)	Genotype 1 SVR (%)	Genotype non-1 SVR (%)
Krawitt [34]	68	PEG IFN α-2b (100–150 μg/week) + RBV 1000 mg daily × 48 weeks[a]	66	54	55	53
Jacobson [35]	25	PEG IFN α-2b 1.0 μg/kg/week + RBV 1000–1200 mg daily × 48 weeks[a]	60	32	27	67
	30	PEG IFN α-2b 1.5 μg/kg/week + RBV 800 mg daily × 48 weeks[a]	77	50	48	60
Gaglio [36]	128	PEG IFN α-2b 1.5 μg/kg/week + RBV 800–1400 mg daily × 48 weeks	78	56	50	60
Portal [38]	24	PEG IFN α-2b 1.5 μg/kg/week + RBV 800–1000 mg daily × 8 weeks, then PEG IFN α-2b 0.7 μg/kg/week + RBV 800–1000 mg daily × 40 weeks	94	69	69	67
	22	PEG IFN α-2b 0.7 μg/kg/week + RBV 800–1000 mg × 48 weeks	88	67	73	50
Lawitz [39]	60	PEG IFN α-2b 1.5 μg/kg/week + RBV 1000–1200 mg daily × 12 weeks, then PEG IFN α-2b 1.0 μg/kg/week + RBV 800 mg daily × 36 weeks	55	30	30	NA
	65	PEG IFN α-2b 1.0 μg/kg/week + RBV 800 mg daily × 48 weeks	58	37	36	NA
Freilich [45]	12	PEG IFN α-2b 1.0 μg/kg/week + RBV 1000 mg daily + AMD 200 mg daily × 48 weeks	NA	50	25	100
	11	PEG IFN α-2b 1.0 μg/kg/week + RBV 1000 mg daily × 48 weeks	NA	36	40	33
Herrine [43]	32	PEG IFN α-2a 180 μg/week + RBV 800–1000 mg daily × 48 weeks	59	38	28	71
	29	PEG IFN α-2a 180 μg/week + MMF 2000 mg daily × 48 weeks	72	17	17	17
	31	PEG IFN α-2a 180 μg/week + AMD 200 mg daily × 48 weeks	42	10	4	20
	31	PEG IFN α-2a 180 μg daily + RBV 800–1000 mg daily + AMD 200 mg daily × 48 weeks	71	45	40	67

Abbreviations: AMD, amantadine; MMF, mycophenolate mofetil.

[a] HCV RNA by PCR was determined at 24 weeks of therapy. If PCR was positive, treatment was discontinued; if PCR was negative, treatment was continued for 48 weeks.

of RBV, and 30 patients were in the group that received the higher dose of IFN. Overall, 69% (38/55) of patients had an end-of-treatment response. Only 42% (23/55), however, had SVR. Thirty-nine percent (15/38) of patients relapsed once therapy was discontinued. There was a trend toward higher SVR rates in patients who received a higher dose of PEG IFN (50% versus 32%), although this difference did not reach statistical significance ($P = 0.18$). SVR rates were lower in genotype 1 patients than in those with other genotypes (38% versus 63%). In this study, patients who were nonresponders to IFN monotherapy or combination IFN and RBV therapy also were treated. SVR rates in prior nonresponders were significantly lower than in patients who had relapsed to therapy previously (8% vs 42%). In a multivariate logistic regression analysis, genotype non-1 and weight greater than 75 kg were associated with high rates of SVR; however, this analysis including both nonresponders and relapsers.

Krawitt et al retreated 68 combination standard IFN and RBV relapsers with a regimen of PEG IFN alfa-2b (100 to 150 μg per week) and ribavirin (1000 mg per day) [34]. In this group of patients, the overall end-of-treatment response rate was 66% (45/68), and the SVR rate was 54% (37/68). Genotype 1 and genotype non-1 patients had similar end-of-treatment (67% and 65%, respectively) and sustained response (55% and 53%) rates. SVR rates were higher in patients who had previously relapsed to therapy than in those who were previous nonresponders. Age and genotype were associated with response rate in previous non-responders but not in relapsers in this study.

Gaglio et al treated patients with PEG IFN alfa-2b (1.5 μg/kg per week) and fixed-dose (800 mg) or weight-based (800 to 1400 mg) RBV for 48 weeks [36]. Of the patients who have completed therapy and reached 24 weeks of follow-up, 78% had an end-of-treatment response, and 56% achieved an SVR. The SVR rate was lower in genotype 1 patients than in those with other genotypes (50% versus 60%). Recently, preliminary data from the lead-in phase of EPIC3, a multicenter study on maintenance therapy with PEG IFN α-2b showed SVR in 39% of relapsers to standard IFN and RBV who were retreated with PEG IFN α-2b (1.5 μg/kg weekly) and weight-based RBV (800 to 1400 mg daily) [37].

In another study by Portal et al in 46 patients, the efficacy of an induction dose of PEG IFN and RBV was compared with a fixed lower dose of PEG IFN and RBV [38]. One group of patients received PEG IFN alfa-2b 1.5 at μg/kg per week plus RBV (800 to 1000 mg per day) for 8 weeks followed by PEG IFN alfa-2b 0.7 μg/kg per week and RBV therapy for 40 weeks. The second group of patients received low-dose PEG IFN alfa-2b 0.7 at μg/kg/week and ribavirin (800 to 100 mg per day) for 48 weeks. The end-of-treatment response rate was 94.1% in the induction group and 88.2% in the group that did not receive induction therapy. SVR rates were similar in both groups (68.7% and 66.7% in the induction and noninduction groups, respectively). SVR rates in this study were unexpectedly higher in patients with genotypes 1 and 4 (69.2% to 72.7%) than in patients with genotypes 2 and 3 (50% to 66.7%). The authors reported that tolerance was similar in both groups, although flu-like symptoms were more frequent in the induction group. The degree of liver fibrosis, as measured by Metavir staging, decreased in approximately 50% percent of patients regardless of the treatment regimen or the ultimate outcome of treatment. In this study, low-dose PEG IFN and RBV therapy was as efficacious as induction-dose therapy.

The efficacy of induction versus fixed-dose PEG IFN and RBV therapy was assessed by Lawitz et al in 125 patients [39]. One group of patients received PEG IFN alfa-2b at 1.5 μg/kg per week and RBV (1000 to 1200 mg per day) for 12 weeks followed by PEG IFN alfa-2b 1.0 μg/kg per week and a reduced dose of RBV (800 mg per day) for 36 weeks. The second group of patients received PEG IFN alfa-2b 1.0 μg/kg per week and RBV (800 mg per day) for 48 weeks. End-of-treatment (58% versus 55%) and sustained virologic response (37% versus 30%) rates were slightly but not significantly higher in the patients receiving induction dosing. Overall SVR rates, as well as SVR rates in patients with genotype 1 with advanced fibrosis (Metavir stage 3-4) were higher in patients who had relapsed after a prior course of therapy than those who were nonresponders to IFN monotherapy or combination IFN and RBV therapy.

Factors predicting sustained virologic response in prior relapsers

In HCV treatment-naïve patients, SVR has been associated with age younger than 40, genotypes 2 and 3, non-African American race, low serum HCV RNA levels (less than 2 million copies/mL), the absence of insulin resistance or steatosis, the absence of bridging fibrosis or cirrhosis, and the absence of coinfection with HIV [40]. During treatment, adherence to therapy and a decline in HCV RNA by greater than 2 logs at 12 weeks of therapy also are associated with achieving an SVR [41,42].

A smaller body of data suggests similar predictors of response in prior relapsers (Box 1). Data on favorable predictors of SVR in prior relapsers are available mostly from patients in studies on relapsers to IFN monotherapy given combination therapy with IFN and RBV; further data on predictors of SVR in combination therapy relapsers given PEG IFN and RBV have recently become available.

In relapsers to IFN monotherapy who are treated, genotype 1 clearly is associated with lower response rates in most studies [20,23,24,29,31,33]. Low pretreatment viral load (less than 2 million copies/mL) [20,23,30,31] and lesser degrees of fibrosis on liver biopsy [23,29,30,33] are predictors of a favorable treatment response, although not all investigators have shown this [19,20,25,27,32]. Older age at treatment and African-American race are associated with poorer response rates [30,31]. Some studies have shown that an elevated ALT level at baseline predicts a favorable response to

Box 1. Predictors of response in prior relapsers:

To standard interferon
- Genotype non-1
- Low viral load
- No or mild fibrosis
- Age greater than 40
- Non-African-American ethnicity
- Early virologic response to therapy

To standard interferon and ribavirin
- Genotype non-1
- Low viral load
- Early virologic response to therapy

antiviral theapy [33]. An early virologic response is also a strong predictor of a virologic cure [20,25].

Longer duration of treatment (24 versus 48 weeks) [22,23,31], particularly for genotype 1 patients with a high viral load, is associated with a better chance for SVR [27,29] in IFN mono-therapy relapsers given IFN and RBV. Higher doses of IFN have not been associated with higher response rates in most studies [23,29,32]. Saracco et al found that the cumulative dose of IFN during the initial course of therapy or retreatment did not predict a favorable response to therapy [29]. Increased dose or duration of therapy in patients with genotypes 2 and 3 is not associated with higher SVR rates [27,29,31].

Similar predictors of response have been recently reported in relapsers to combination standard IFN and RBV therapy who are retreated with PEG IFN and RBV. Genotype non-1 and low viral load are predictors of a favorable response [43,44]. In one study, the absence of HCV viremia at week 6, as determined by the transcription-mediated amplification assay, was highly predictive of SVR (80% in the overall study population, 92% in genotype non-1 patients) [44].

Adjunctive therapies for patients who have relapsed after interferon and ribavirin combination therapy

In an effort to improve SVR rates in this population, some investigators have evaluated adjunctive therapies in addition to PEG IFN α2b and RBV. Freilich et al assessed the benefit of adding amantadine to PEG IFN and RBV therapy in treating patients who previously had relapsed to therapy [45]. They compared PEG IFN (1.0 μg/kg per week) and RBV (1000 mg per day) with a regimen of PEG IFN (1.0 μg/kg per week) and RBV (1000 mg per day) plus amantadine (200 mg per day). The overall SVR rate presented from interim data in 23 patients was 43%. The addition of amantadine was not beneficial in genotype 1 relapsers. The SVR rate in genotype 1 relapsers was 25% (2/8) in patients treated with amantadine and 40% (2/5) in those treated with standard PEG IFN and RBV combination therapy. In contrast, the addition of amantadine may have led to superior treatment efficacy in nongenotype 1 patients. All (4/4) of the genotype non-1 patients treated with amantadine had an SVR, compared with only 33% (two of six) of patients treated with PEG IFN and RBV alone, but final data from this study are not available, and the number of patients is too small to draw any definitive conclusions.

In another study, 37 relapsers (to standard IFN monotherapy or standard IFN and RBV combination therapy) were retreated with an induction dose of standard IFN (18 MU daily) in combination with ribavirin (1000 to 1200 mg daily) and amantadine (100 mg daily) for two weeks and then randomized to 22 weeks of continued ribavirin and amantadine with or without IFN (6 MU three times weekly) [44]. The 10 patients who discontinued interferon after the 2 week induction course all relapsed within two weeks. Of the patients who received 24 weeks of interferon, the end-of-treatment response was 63% (17/27) and the SVR rate was 44% (12/27). Twenty nine percent (5/17) of patients with an end-of-treatment response subsequently relapsed.

Herrine et al assessed the efficacy of mycophenolate mofetil and amantadine in addition to PEG IFN and RBV in a pilot study [43]. They treated 124 patients (106 relapsers, 18 breakthrough relapsers) who were randomized to receive PEG IFN alfa-2a 180 μg once weekly in addition to one of four following treatment arms: (1) RBV at 800 to 1000 mg daily, (2) mycophenolate at 1000 mg twice daily, (3) amantadine at 100 mg twice daily, or (4) amantadine at 100 mg twice daily and RBV at 800 to 1000 mg daily. End-of-treatment response rates were highest in patients who were treated with PEG IFN and mycophenolate (72.4%) and PEG IFN, RBV, and amantadine (71%). Patients who received PEG IFN, RBV, and amantadine had the highest SVR rates (45%), followed by those who received PEG IFN and RBV (38%). However, the difference in response rates in the two groups did not reach statistical significance. Treatment with PEG IFN and either amantadine or mycophenolate alone resulted in lower SVR rates (10% and 17%, respectively), as in other trials. Thus, RBV appears to exact its benefit by preventing relapse. There was a trend towards higher SVR rates in patients with genotype non-1 and low HCV viral load. Tolerance of the medications was similar in the different treatment groups, except for the more significant decline in hemoglobin seen in patients who received ribavirin.

Approach to the retreatment of patients who relapse after interferon and ribavirin combination therapy

Patients who relapse after standard IFN and RBV should be considered strongly for retreatment with PEG IFN and RBV because of their significant chance of SVR (30% to 70%). The available data are derived from studies in which PEG IFN and RBV were administered for 48 weeks. In these studies, however, relapse even after PEG IFN and RBV occurred in significant numbers of patients. Current viral kinetic models suggest that a gradual second phase of HCV-infected cell death occurs, ultimately leading to viral eradication in patients who achieve an SVR [17]. It is thought that patients who relapse may have a more prolonged period of elimination of infected cells, which may not have been completed when a standard course of IFN and RBV therapy ends. Therefore, in these patients with a previously demonstrated proclivity to relapse, longer courses of therapy than the standard duration of 48 weeks may be worth consideration in the retreatment of selected patients, with a goal of maximizing the chance of eventual eradication of all virally infected cells. Such patients might include those with genotype 1, high viral load, and advanced fibrosis, or those with a delayed response to therapy. However, controlled trials demonstrating the efficacy of such prolonged therapy have not been reported.

Adherence to optimal doses of PEG IFN and RBV during prior therapy also should be considered. The superior efficacy (44% versus 41%, $P = 0.02$) of weight-based (800 mg to 1400 mg) versus fixed (800 mg) RBV dosing has been recently demonstrated in a multicenter, randomized, community based trial of 4913 patients [46]. In treatment naïve patients, dose reductions of either drug, and particularly both drugs, have a significant impact on attainment of early virologic response (EVR) after 12 weeks (80% EVR with full doses versus 60% to 70% and 33% with dose reduction of either or both drugs, respectively) [47]. In patients who attain EVR, the chance of SVR is adversely affected by dose reductions or discontinuation of therapy beyond the 12-week timepoint. Although comparable data do not exist for the relapse population, these same principles may well apply. Accordingly, every effort must be made to maintain optimal dosing during the retreatment of patients who have relapsed to a prior course of therapy. Patients who underwent dose reduction during prior therapy for depression, anemia, or neutropenia may be considered for antidepressants, granulocyte colony stimulating factor therapy, or erythropoietin, respectively, as appropriate during retreatment. It must be recognized, however, that while recent studies on erythropoietin show an effect on successful maintenance of ribavirin dose, improvements in hemoglobin levels and quality of life [48], no prospective trials have demonstrated the use of adjunctive factors to enhance SVR.

Treatment of patients who have relapsed after pegylated interferon and ribavirin combination therapy

Patients who have relapsed after a course of PEG IFN and RBV pose a difficult problem, because more effective therapy is not available. There are no data on the efficacy of higher doses of drugs, leaving a repeat course of more prolonged therapy as the major option. Goncales et al treated naïve patients with either 24 or 48 weeks of combination PEG IFN alfa-2a and RBV. Patients who received 24 weeks of therapy and relapsed were eligible to enter a retreatment study consisting of PEG IFN alfa-2a (maximum dose of 180 μg per week) and RBV (1000 to 12000 mg per day) for 48 weeks [49]. PEG IFN and RBV doses were adjusted by the investigators according to the patients' tolerance of the medications during the initial course of therapy. Preliminary data from this study on 59 patients indicate high end of treatment virologic response rates of 90% (88% in genotype 1 patients; 93% in patients with genotype 2 and 3) with retreatment. SVR rates from this study are awaited.

Because most patients who relapse after a course of PEG IFN and RBV will have received 48 weeks of therapy, the only realistic option is to consider a repeat course of treatment for a longer duration (eg, 72 to 96 weeks). In apparent conformity with concepts of the kinetics of viral clearance, patients who clear HCV RNA on their initial course of PEG IFN and RBV have an enhanced risk of post-treatment relapse if clearance of HCV RNA requires longer than 12 weeks of therapy [41]. The concept of modifying the duration of therapy according to a patient's virologic response pattern to PEG IFN and RBV therapy has been evaluated in a preliminary study of nine HCV genotype 1, treatment-naïve patients [50]. These nine patients all had delayed virologic clearance; they were positive for HCV RNA by PCR but had a 2 log decline in HCV RNA by week 12 of therapy and had cleared virus by week 24. Patients were treated for 72 weeks, and 88% (7/8, with one lost to follow-up) had an SVR. As in patients with relapse after a course of standard IFN and RBV, this approach to therapy needs to be evaluated further in patients who have relapsed after a prior course of PEG IFN and RBV, particularly patients with genotype 1, high viral load, and cirrhosis, or patients in whom clearance of HCV RNA was delayed beyond 12 weeks.

Preliminary data with consensus interferon, a novel recombinant type 1 interferon, suggests sustained virologic response rates of 23–37% in previous nonresponders to pegylated interferon and ribavirin [51,52]. However, data from large multicenter studies is needed to confirm these findings in prior nonresponders. Studies evaluating the efficacy of consensus interferon in prior relapsers to PEG IFN and RBV are currently in progress, including at our center.

Future directions

In addition to the options of PEG IFN and RBV for relapsers to previous combination therapy, or prolonged courses of PEG IFN and RBV in relapsers to previous PEG IFN and RBV therapy, new therapies on the horizon for treatment-naïve patients with chronic hepatitis C include genome sequence-based therapies, viral enzyme inhibitors, and immunomodulatory agents may be efficacious in patients who have relapsed to previous therapy also [9,53]. Most promising are the protease and polymerase inhibitors which are currently in Phase I and Phase II trials. Preliminary data from both treatment-naïve HCV-infected patients and previous nonresponders have demonstrated marked declines in HCV viremia with these novel compounds [54–57]. Patients with mild liver disease or those who had great difficulty tolerating interferon-based therapy may wish to defer retreatment as novel therapies are awaited. In the authors' practice, however, it is felt that most patients with relapse after standard IFN and RBV should be offered a course of PEG IFN and RBV.

Summary

Sustained virologic response rates are significantly higher in patients who have relapsed after a previous course of therapy compared with patients who did not respond. A meta-analysis of combination therapy in patients who failed IFN monotherapy reported SVR rates of 52% in relapsers to prior therapy and 16% in nonresponders [12]. Similarly, relapsers after combination standard IFN and RBV therapy have higher SVR rates than combination of therapy nonresponders when treated with pegylated interferon and ribavirin [34,35–39]. For this reason, patients who relapse after a previous course of therapy should be considered potential candidates for retreatment. Factors that have been associated with SVR in these patients include genotype non-1, low viral loads, and lesser degrees of fibrosis. The course of treatment in all patients who have relapsed after prior therapy should be reviewed to identify possible reasons for failure to achieve an SVR. In particular, optimal dosing of PEG IFN and RBV and the occurrence and timing of treatment dose reductions during prior therapy should be reviewed. The reasons for dose reduction should be addressed before initiating another course of therapy in an effort to optimize the chance for a SVR. Patients who had dose reduction for depression, anemia, or neutropenia, should be considered for antidepressants, erythropoietin, or, if neutropenia is severe, granulocyte colony stimulating factor therapy, respectively, during retreatment. Prolongation of therapy beyond 48 weeks in patients with relapse after a standard course of PEG IFN and RBV may offer a chance of SVR. Novel agents currently in development, including protease and polymerase inhibitors, may prove to be therapeutic options for these patients in the future.

References

[1] Poynard T, Marcellin P, Lee SS, Niederau C, Minuk GS, Ideo G, et al. Randomised trial of interferon α2b plus ribavirin for 48 weeks or for 24 weeks versus interferon α2b plus placebo for 48 weeks for treatment of chronic infection with hepatitis C virus. Lancet 1998;352: 1426–32.

[2] McHutchison JG, Gordon SC, Schiff ER, Shiffman ML, Lee WM, Rustgi VK, et al. Interferon alfa-2b alone or in combination with ribavirin as initial treatment for chronic hepatitis C. N Engl J Med 1998;339:1485–92.

[3] Lau JYN, Tam RC, Liang TJ, Hong Z. Mechanisms of action of ribavirin in the combination treatment of chronic HCV infection. Hepatology 2002;35(5):1002–9.
[4] Graci JD, Cameron CE. Quasispecies, error catastrophe, and the antiviral activity of ribavirin. Virology 2002;298:175–80.
[5] Dixit NM, Layden-Almer JE, Layden TJ, et al. Modelling how ribavirin improves interferon response rates in hepatitis C virus infection. Nature 2004;432:922–4.
[6] Dusheiko G, Main J, Thomas H, Reichard O, Lee C, Dhillon A, et al. Ribavirin treatment for patients with chronic hepatitis C: results of a placebo-controlled study. J Hepatol 1996; 25:591–8.
[7] Di Bisceglie AM, Shindo M, Fong TL, Fried MW, Swain MG, Bergasa NV, et al. A pilot study of ribavirin therapy for chronic hepatitis C. Hepatology 1992;16:649–54.
[8] Bodenheimer HC Jr, Lindsay KL, Davis GL, Lewis JH, Thung SN, Seef LB. Tolerance and efficacy of oral ribavirin treatment of chronic hepatitis C: A multi-center trial. Hepatology 1997;26:473–7.
[9] Brouwer JT, Nevens F, Bekkering FC, et al. Reduction of relapse rates by 18-month treatment in chronic hepatitis C. A Benelux randomized trial in 300 patients. J Hepatol 2004;40: 689–95.
[10] Manns MP, McHutchison JG, Gordon SC, Rustgi VK, Shiffman M, Reindollar R, et al. Peginterferon alfa-2b plus ribavirin compared with interferon alfa-2b plus ribavirin for the initial treatment of chronic hepatitis C: a randomised trial. Lancet 2001;358:958–65.
[11] Fried MW, Shiffman ML, Reddy R, Smith C, Marinos G, Goncales FL, et al. Peginterferon alfa-2a plus ribavirin for chronic hepatitis C virus infection. N Engl J Med 2002;347(13): 975–82.
[12] Poynard T, McHutchison J, Manns M, et al. Impact of pegylated interferon alfa-2b and ribavirin on liver fibrosis in patients with chronic hepatitis C. Gastroenterology 2002;122: 1303–13.
[13] Coverdale SA, Khan MH, Byth K, et al. Effects of interferon treatment response in liver complications of chronic hepatitis C: 9-year follow-up study. Am J Gastroenterol 2004; 99(4):636–44.
[14] Davis GL, Lau JYN. Factors predictive of a beneficial response to therapy of hepatitis C. Hepatology 1997;26(3):S122–7.
[15] Leroy V, Baud M, de Traversay C, Maynard-Muet M, Lebon P, Zarski JP. Role of anti-interferon antibodies in breakthrough occurrence during alpha 2a and 2b therapy in patients with chronic hepatitis C. J Hepatol 1998;28(3):375–81.
[16] Hoffmann RM, Berg T, Teuber G, Prummer O, Leifeld L, Jung MC, et al. Interferon antibodies and the breakthrough phenomenon during ribavirin/interferon-alpha combination therapy and interferon-alpha monotherapy of patients with chronic hepatitis. Z Gastroenterol 1999;37(8):715–23.
[17] Neumann AU, Lam NP, Dahari H, Gretch DR, Wiley TE, Layden TJ, et al. Hepatitis C viral dynamics in vivo and the antiviral efficacy of interferon-α therapy. Science 1998;282: 103–7.
[18] Sarrazin C, Teuber G, Kokka R, et al. Detection of residual hepatitis C virus RNA by transcription-mediated amplification in patients with complete virologic response according to polymerase chain reaction-based assays. Hepatology 2000;32:818–23.
[19] Chow WC, Boyer N, Pouteau M, Castelnau C, Martinot-Peignoux M, Martins-Amado V, et al. Re-treatment with interferon alfa of patients with chronic hepatitis C. Hepatology 1998;27:1144–8.
[20] Davis GL, Esteban-Mur R, Rustgi V, Hoefs J, Gordon SC, Trepo C, et al. Interferon alfa-2b alone or in combination with ribavirin for the treatment of relapse of chronic hepatitis C. N Engl J Med 1998;339:1493–9.
[21] Weiland O, Zhang YY, Widell A. Serum HCV RNA levels in patients with chronic hepatitis C given a second course of interferon alpha-2b treatment after relapse following initial treatment. Scand J Infect Dis 1993;25:25–30.

[22] Picciotto A, Brizzolara R, Campo N, Poggi G, Sinelli N, De Conca V, et al. Two-year interferon retreatment may induce a sustained response in relapsing patients with chronic hepatitis C. Hepatology 1996;24(4):273A.

[23] Payen JL, Izopet J, Galindo-Migeot V, Lauwers-Cances V, Zarski JP, Seigneurin JM, et al. Better efficacy of a 12-month interferon alfa-2b retreatment in patients with chronic hepatitis C relapsing after a 6-month treatment: a multi-center, controlled, randomized trial. Hepatology 1998;28:1680–6.

[24] Bell H, Hellum K, Harthug S, Myrvang B, Ritland S, Maeland A, et al. Treatment with interferon-alpha 2a alone or interferon-alpha 2a plus ribavirin in patients with chronic hepatitis C previously treated with interferon-alpha 2a. Scand J Gastroenterol 1999;34: 194–8.

[25] Barbaro G, Di Lorenzo G, Belloni G, Ferrari L, Paiano A, Del Poggio P, et al. Interferon alpha-2b and ribavirin in combination for patients with chronic hepatitis C who failed to respond to, or relapsed after, interferon alpha therapy: a randomized trial. Am J Med 1999; 107:112–8.

[26] Cavalletto L, Chemello L, Donada C, Casarin P, Belussi F, Bernardinello E, et al. The pattern of response to interferon alpha (α-IFN) predicts sustained response to a 6-month α-IFN and ribavirin retreatment for chronic hepatitis C. J Hepatol 2000;33:128–34.

[27] Enriquez J, Gallego A, Torras X, Perez-Olmeda T, Diago M, Soriano V, et al. Retreatment for 24 vs 48 weeks with interferon-α2b plus ribavirin of chronic hepatitis C patients who relapsed or did not respond to interferon alone. J Viral Hepat 2000;7:403–8.

[28] Cozzolongo R, Cuppone R, Giannuzzi V, Amati L, Caradonna L, Tamborrino V, et al. Combination therapy with ribavirin and alpha interferon for the treatment of chronic hepatitis C refractory to interferon. Alimentary Pharmacology and Therapeutics 2001;15: 129–35.

[29] Saracco G, Olivero A, Ciancio A, Carenzi S, Smedile A, Cariti G, et al. A randomized 4-arm multi-center study of interferon alfa-2b plus ribavirin in the treatment of patients with chronic hepatitis C relapsing after interferon monotherapy. Hepatology 2002;36: 959–66.

[30] Shiffman ML, Hoofmann CM, Sterling RK, Luketic VA, Contos MJ, Sanyal AJ. A randomized, controlled trial to determine whether continued ribavirin monotherapy in hepatitis C virus-infected patients who responded to interferon–ribavirin combination therapy will enhance sustained virologic response. J Infect Dis 2001;184:405–9.

[31] Di Marco V, Almasio P, Vaccaro A, Ferraro A, Parisi P, Cataldo MG, et al. Combined treatment of relapse of chronic hepatitis C with high-dose α_2b interferon plus ribavirin for 6 to 12 months. J Hepatol 2000;33:456–62.

[32] Min AD, Jones JL, Esposito S, Lebovics E, Jacobson IM, Klion FM, et al. Efficacy of high-dose interferon in combination with ribavirin in patients with chronic hepatitis C resistant to interferon alone. Am J Gastroenterol 2001;96(4):1143–9.

[33] Portal I, Bourliere M, Halfon P, et al. Retreatment with interferon and ribavirin vs interferon alone according to viraemia in interferon responder-relapser hepatitis C patients: a prospective multicentre randomized controlled study. J Viral Hepatitis 2003;10:215–23.

[34] Krawitt EL, Ashikaga T, Gordon SR, et al. Peginterferon alfa-2b and ribavirin for treatment-refractory chronic hepatitis C. J Hepatol 2005;43:243–9.

[35] Jacobson IM, Gonzalez SA, Ahmed F, et al. A randomized trial of pegylated interferon α-2b plus ribavirin in the retreatment of chronic hepatitis C. Am J Gastroenterol 2005;100:1–10.

[36] Gaglio P, Choi J, Zimmerman D, et al. Weight based ribavirin in combination with pegylated interferon alpha 2-b does not improve SVR in HCV infected patients who failed prior therapy: results in 454 patients. Hepatology 2005;42(4, suppl 1):219A.

[37] Poynard T, Schiff E, Terg R, et al. Sustained virologic response (SVR) with PEG-interferon-alfa-2b/ribavirin weight based dosing in previous interferon/ribavirin HCV treatment failures; week 12 virology as a predictor of SVR in the EPIC3 trials. Gastroenterology 2005; 128:A681.

[38] Portal I, Botta-Fridlund D, Bourliere M, Couzigou P, Barange K, Canva V, et al. Treatment with pegylated-interferon alpha-2b (peg-interferon) + ribavirin in relapsers to standard interferon + ribavirin in chronic hepatitis C: efficacy and safety results from a randomized multi-centric French study. Hepatology 2002;36(4):359A.
[39] Lawitz EJ, Bala NS, Becker S, Brown G, Davis M, Dhar R, et al. Pegylated interferon alfa 2b and ribavirin for hepatitis C patients who were nonresponders to previous therapy. Gastroenterology 2003;124(4):A783.
[40] Ferenci P. Predictors of response to therapy for chronic hepatitis C. Seminars in Liver Disease 2004;24(Suppl 2):25–31.
[41] Davis GL, Wong JB, McHutchison JG, Mann MP, Harvey J, Albrecht J, et al. Early virologic response to treatment with pegylated interferon α-2b and ribavirin in patients with chronic hepatitis C. Hepatology 2003;38:645–52.
[42] McHutchison JG, Manns M, Patel K, Poynard T, Lindsay KL, Trepo C, et al. Adherence to combination therapy enhances sustained response in genotype-1 infected patients with chronic hepatitis C. Gastroenterology 2002;123:1061–9.
[43] Herrine SK, Brown RS, Bernstein DE, et al. Peginterferon α-2a combination therapies in chronic hepatitis C patients who relapsed after or had a viral breakthrough on therapy with standard interferon α-2b plus ribavirin: a pilot study of efficacy and safety. Dig Dis Sci 2005;50(4):719–26.
[44] Weegink CJ, Sentjens RE, Beld MG, et al. Chronic hepatitis C patients with a post-treatment virological relapse re-treated with an induction dose of 18 MU interferon-α in combination with ribavirin and amantadine: a two-arm randomized pilot study. J Viral Hepatol 2003;10: 174–82.
[45] Freilich B, Weston A, DeGuzmann LJ, Kissinger J. Triple therapy for interferon/ribavirin failure patients with hepatitis C: interim data. Hepatology 2002;36(4):361A.
[46] Jacobson IM, Brown RS, Freilich B, et al. Weight-based ribavirin dosing (WBD) increases sustained viral response (SVR) in patients with chronic hepatitis C (CHC): final results of the WIN-R study, a US community based trial. Hepatology 2005;42(4, Suppl 1):749A.
[47] Davis GL, Wong JB, McHutchison JG, et al. Early virologic response to treatment with peginterferon alfa-2b plus ribavirin in patients with chronic hepatitis C. Hepatology 2003;38: 645–52.
[48] Afdhal NH, Dieterich DT, Pockros PJ, et al. Epoetin alfa maintains ribavirin dose in HCV-infected patients: a prospective, double-blind, randomized controlled study. Gastroenterology 2004;126:1302–11.
[49] Goncales F, Berstein DE, Berg C, Sette H, Rasenack J, Diago M, et al. Peginterferon alfa-2a (40KD) (Pegasys) plus ribavirin in chronic hepatitis C: retreatment of patients who relapsed virologically after 24 weeks of therapy. Hepatology 2002;36(4):361A.
[50] Buti M, Valdes A, Sanchez-Avila F, Esteban R, Lurie Y. Extending combination therapy with peginterferon alfa-2b plus ribavirin for genotype 1 chronic hepatitis C late responders: a report of 9 cases. Hepatology 2003;37(5):1226–7.
[51] Leevey CB, Chalmers CP, Blatt LM. Comparison of African American and Non-African American patient end of treatment response for Peg-IFN α-2 and weight-based ribavirin nonresponders re-treated with IFN alfacon-1 and weight-based ribavirin. Hepatology 2004;40(4, Suppl 1):240A.
[52] Kaiser S, Hass H, Gregor. Successful retreatment of chronic hepatitis C patients with a non-response to standard interferon/ribavirin using daily consensus interferon and ribavirin. Hepatology 2004;40(4, Suppl 1):240A.
[53] Di Bisceglie AM, McHutchison JG, Rice CM. New therapeutic strategies for hepatitis C. Hepatology 2002;35(1):224–31.
[54] Zeuzem S, Sarrazin C, Rouzier R, Tarral A, Brion N, Forestier N, et al. Anti-viral activity of SCH 503034, a HCV protease inhibitor, administered as monotherapy in hepatitis C genotype-1 (HCV-1) patients refractory to pegylated interferon (PEG-IFN-α). Hepatology 2005; 42(4, Suppl 1):233A–4A.

[55] Reesink HW, Zeuzem S, Weegink CJ, Forestier N, van VLiet A, ven de Wetering de Rooij J, et al. Final results of a phase 1B, multiple-dose study of VX-950, a hepatitis C virus protease inhibitor. Hepatology 2005;42(4, Suppl 1):234A–5A.
[56] O'Brien C, Godofsky E, Rodriguez-Torres M, Afdhal N, Pappas SC, Pockros P, et al. Randomized trial of valopicitabine (NM283), alone or in with PEG-interferon, vs. retreatment with PEG-interferon plus ribavirin (PEGIFN/RBV) in hepatitis C patients with previous nonresponse to PEGIFN/RBV: first interim results. Hepatology 2005;42(4, Suppl 1):234A.
[57] Sarisky RT. Non-nucleoside inhibitors of the HCV polymerase. Journal of Antimicrobial Chemotherapy 2004;54:14–6.

ELSEVIER
SAUNDERS

Infect Dis Clin N Am
20 (2006) 155–174

INFECTIOUS
DISEASE CLINICS
OF NORTH AMERICA

Management of Recurrent Hepatitis C in Liver Transplant Recipients

Scott W. Biggins, MD, Norah A. Terrault, MD, MPH*

Division of Gastroenterology, Department of Medicine, University of California, San Francisco, 513 Parnassus Ave, S357, Box 0538 San Francisco, CA 94143, USA

Chronic hepatitis C virus (HCV) infection is the most common indication for liver transplantation in the United States and Europe, and more than 20,000 patients worldwide have undergone transplantation for complications of chronic hepatitis C. In North America, HCV accounts for 15% to 50% of all liver transplants performed [1]. Available prevalence data predict that this proportion will likely increase as the number of persons with chronic hepatitis C developing cirrhosis and hepatocellular carcinoma in North America rises over the next 1 to 2 decades [2,3].

Recurrent HCV infection is universal in those with viremia before transplantation, and the rate of histologic disease progression after transplantation is more rapid. The risk of death and allograft failure is increased in HCV-positive transplant recipients (hazard ratio [HR] 1.23 and 1.30) compared with HCV-negative recipients [4]. The risk of cirrhosis is as high as 30% within 5 to 10 years after transplantation [5–7]. Retransplantation for recurrent hepatitis C is an option for only a limited number of patients, and with a 5-year survival rate of $\leq$ 50%, it is likely to remain a controversial indication for retransplantation [8].

To maximize the long-term survival of liver transplant recipients who have HCV infection, eradication of infection is the ultimate goal. Pretransplant antiviral therapy with the goal of achieving viral eradication before transplantation is a consideration in some patients, especially those who have mildly decompensated liver disease [9]. This article focuses on the management of liver transplant recipients who have HCV infection at the time of transplantation. This group of patients is at risk for recurrent and progressive disease after transplantation. There are several different time points for

A version of this article originally appeared in the 9:3 issue of Clinics in Liver Disease.

* Corresponding author.
E-mail address: Norah.Terrault@ucsf.edu (N.A. Terrault).

doi:10.1016/j.idc.2006.01.011 *id.theclinics.com*

considering treatment interventions (Fig. 1): (1) Prophylactic therapy is started prior to or at the time of transplantation and continued for variable periods post-transplant. The goal of prophylaxis is to prevent reinfection of the graft. (2) Preemptive therapy of recurrent HCV infection refers to initiation of therapy early in the post-transplant period, typically within the first 4 to 8 weeks after transplantation, and before biochemical and histologic disease are manifest. (3) Therapy for established recurrent disease refers to the use of antiviral treatment when there is biochemical and histologic evidence of recurrent disease. Treatment of established recurrent disease has been the most frequently used strategy for the management of post-transplant HCV infection.

Natural history of recurrent hepatitis C virus after transplantation

Recurrent infection, defined by the presence of detectable HCV RNA in serum and liver, occurs in essentially all patients who are viremic pretransplant. Kinetic studies of the early virologic events after transplantation have shown that HCV RNA levels drop abruptly during the anhepatie phase and again 8 to 24 hours after reperfusion [10]. In general, viral levels increase beginning 24 to 72 hours post-transplant, but there is considerable interpatient variability in the rate of increase in viral levels during the first postoperative week [10]. Thereafter, a progressive increase in viral load occurs in the majority of patients, with the peak viral level occurring between months 1 and 4 [11]. At 1 year post-transplant, HCV RNA levels are on average 1-$\log_{10}$ higher than pretransplant levels [12,13]. Pretransplant viral liters have been inconsistently correlated with post-transplant HCV RNA levels [13]. High pretransplant viral levels have been associated with reduced overall

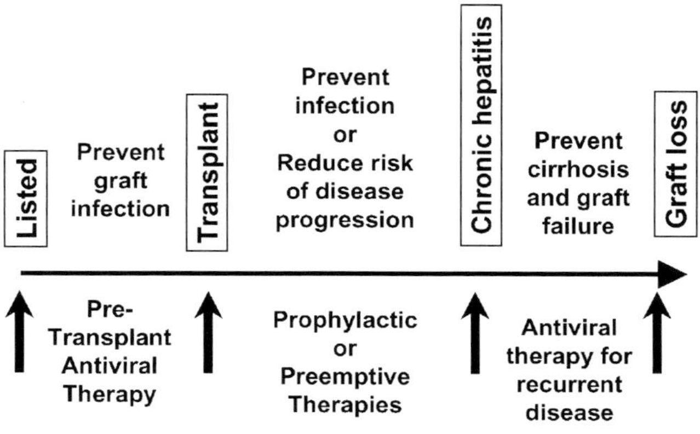

Fig. 1. This identifies the potential time points for intervening with therapy to prevent or eradicate HCV infection or slow disease progression. (Courtesy of M Berenguer, MD, Valencia, Spain.)

patient and graft survival in one study [14], but whether this reflects the effects of HCV recurrence per se or other transplant complications to which HCV-infected persons with high pretransplant levels of HCV are more susceptible is unknown, HCV genotype has not been found to be predictive of post-transplant HCV RNA levels. Multiple studies have shown post-transplant HCV viral liters to correlate poorly with histologic severity of disease [15–17].

Histologic manifestations of recurrent hepatitis C are variable, but the majority of patients have evidence of chronic hepatitis on liver biopsy within the first year. Approximately 70% develop acute hepatitis, usually within the first 3 to 6 months after transplantation, which evolves to chronic hepatitis. Chronic hepatitis without a preceding acute hepatitis occurs in about 20% of patients and may have a more favorable outcome in terms of disease progression. A severe and rapidly progressive form of recurrent disease, termed cholestatic hepatitis, is associated with a histologic pattern of ballooned hepatocytes, confluent necrosis, bile duct proliferation, and cholestasis, but with minimal inflammation [18]. Another hallmark of cholestatic hepatitis is high serum HCV RNA levels ($>10^6$ IU/mL) [19]. Historically, the outcome of cholestatic hepatitis was dismal, with mortality rates of 50% within the first year. This severe manifestation of recurrent disease occurs in 10% or less of HCV-infected transplant recipients, and antiviral therapy has been recently shown to result in disease stabilization and prolonged survival in some recipients with this condition [20,21].

Fibrosis progression in liver transplant recipients is more rapid than in nontransplant patients. In untreated patients, 8% to 44% develop recurrent cirrhosis within 5 to 7 years of transplantation [5–7,22–24]. Once cirrhosis develops, the risk of decompensation and graft loss are high, with one study reporting 42% mortality within 1 year [25]. Another study suggested the rate of fibrosis progression was not linear. Mean fibrosis scores were 1.2 after 1 year, 1.7 after 3 years, 1.9 after 5 years, 2.1 after 7 years, and 2.2 after 10 years [26]. Several studies indicate that early aggressive disease carries a worse prognosis [13,23,26]. Patients with high histologic activity within the first year post-transplant are at greatest risk of progressive fibrosis and cirrhosis. One study found the presence of confluent necrosis on early biopsy to be highly predictive of risk of cirrhosis [26]. In a recent study, 39 recipients with fibrosis stages 3 or 4 at the 1-year biopsy had a significantly reduced survival compared with those with stages 0 to 2 at 1 year [23].

Factors associated with severity of hepatitis C virus recurrence

Numerous studies have sought to identify recipient, donor, viral, and other factors that are associated with severe and progressive recurrent hepatitis C. End points for these studies differ, with some studies focused on fibrosis progression or incidence of cirrhosis and others using graft or patient survival as a marker of severe disease outcome (Table 1). Analysis of survival rather than histology may lead to overestimation of graft and patient losses due to HCV because other causes of graft loss (eg, chronic rejection) and non–liver-related causes of death (eg, sepsis) are included. Additionally, the predictors of "all causes" graft survival may not mirror those of progressive HCV disease leading to graft loss.

One of the more controversial factors linked with more severe HCV disease is the use of a living donor. Theoretically, the rapid regeneration of the living donor graft in the postoperative period may alter early virologic or immunologic events related to HCV recurrence such that disease progression is more rapid. Live donors are also more likely to share human leukocyte antigens, which may alter the natural history of post-transplant recurrence. Studies using graft survival as the primary outcome are difficult

Table 1
Possible factors associated with increased severity of hepatitis C virus recurrence

Study	Donor factors	Recipient factors	HCV-specific factors	Other factors
Worse graft and patient survival				
Charlton, 1998 [14]	—	—	HCV RNA >1 MEq/mL at transplantation	—
Berenguer, 2002 [37]	Donor age	Female gender	—	Year of LT OKT3 induction
Burak, 2002 [34]	—	—	—	CMV infection
Sanchez-Fueyo, 2002 [6]	—	—	Biochemical hepatitis	CMV disease
Neumann, 2004 [23]	Donor age	—	Genotype 1 and 4	Number of steroid boluses
Thuluvath, 2004 [27]	LD	—	—	—
Garcia-Retortillo, 2004 [32]	LD	—	—	—
More advanced histological fibrosis				
Berenguer, 2000 [5]	—	Non-white race	HCV RNA at LT	Year of LT Number of corticosteroid boluses
Papatheodoridis, 2001 [35]	—	—	—	Triple or dual versus single initial IMS
Berenguer, 2002 [37]	Donor age	—	Acute recurrent hepatitis	OKT3 induction TAC induction
Burak, 2002 [34]	Donor age	Recipient age	—	Year of LT CMV infection MMF use
Guido, 2002 [26]	—	—	Severity of necroinflammation within first year	—

Abbreviations: CMV, cytomegalovirus; HCV, hepatitis C virus; IMS, immunosuppression; LD, live donor graft; LT, liver transplantation; MMF, mycophenolate mofetil; TAC, tacrolimus.

to interpret because the complications related to live donor liver transplantation per se may be the cause of worse outcome rather than more severe recurrent hepatitis C. This was shown in a study of 764 live donor liver transplant (LDLT) and 1470 matched deceased donor liver transplant (DDLT) recipients, with 2-year graft survival rates of 64% and 73%, respectively ($P < .001$) [27]. Among LDLT recipients, the risk of graft failure was 60% higher (HR 1.6, 95% confidence interval [CI] 1.1–2.5) after adjusting for baseline differences in the groups such as serum creatinine, United Network of Organ Sharing (UNOS) status, and need for life support [27]. Similar to the overall analysis, a subanalysis of HCV-positive patients found graft survival to be lower in LDLT compared with DDLT recipients. A second study of UNOS data by Russo and colleagues [28] found no significant difference in survival between 279 LDLT and 3955 DDLT recipients who were HCV positive, with 2-year graft survival rates of 72% and 75%, respectively ($P = .11$). Six studies have been published on this issue, with no differences in outcome between LDLT and DDLT recipients reported in four of six studies (Table 2) [29]. The rate of cholestatic hepatitis was significantly higher (17% versus 0%) in live donor versus deceased donor recipients in one single-center study [30], but the time to recurrence and overall severity of disease was not different between groups. Only two studies have used protocol biopsies to assess for HCV disease recurrence and progression and are most informative in terms of the effect of donor type on HCV natural history. In a United States study of 23 LDLT and 53 DDLT patients, patient and graft survival was not different, and there was no patient with cirrhosis in either group at the end of a median 40 months follow-up [31]. In a Spanish study of similar study design, results were different. Cirrhosis or liver decompensation occurred in 44% of LDLT patients, compared with 29% of DDLT patients ($P = .019$) [32]. With these divergent results, no definite conclusion can be drawn. Although there is no rationale for HCV-positive patients to be denied access to a timely transplant if a liver donor is available, physicians should discuss with patients the unclear impact of LDLT on HCV disease progression.

The factors most consistently associated with a high risk of progression to cirrhosis and graft loss due to HCV infection include treated acute rejection, cytomegalovirus infection, nonwhite race, and early severe or acute recurrence. Corticosteroid boluses, cumulative corticosteroid doses, and the use of lymphocyte-depleting agents have been associated with increased HCV RNA levels and are linked with progressive HCV disease in some studies [33].

The relationship between other immunosuppressive agents and severity of HCV disease progression after transplantation are even less clear (Table 3). Steroid-free immunosuppressive regimens have shown some benefits in HCV-infected recipients [34]. Retrospective analyses of patients receiving tacrolimus versus cyclosporine-based immunosuppression show no difference in disease severity between calcineurin inhibitor groups [35,36,37]. The impact

Table 2
Comparison of live donor and deceased donor liver transplant recipients with hepatitis C

Study	Study population	*n* (LD/DD)	Mean follow-up time (mo)	Outcomes
Gaglio, 2003 [30]	Single center	23/45	26	No difference in graft survival, time to recurrence, or incidence of recurrence Higher rate of cholestatic hepatitis in LDLT versus DDLT (17% versus 0%)
Shiffman, 2004 [31]	Single center	23/53	40	No difference in graft survival: 82% and 82% at 2 yr
Russo, 2004 [28]	UNOS	279/3955	—	No difference in graft survival at 2 yr, LDLT versus DDLT (72% versus 75%)
Thuluvath, 2004 [27]	UNOS	764/1470	—	Worse graft survival at 2 yr for LDLT versus DDLT (64% versus 73%) (OR 1.6, 95% CI 1.1–2.5)
Bozorgzadeh, 2004 [29]	Single center	35/65	25	No difference in graft survival at 39 months for LDLT versus DDLT (72% versus 64%)
Garcia-Retortillo, 2004 [32]	Single center	22/95	22	Increased probability of severe recurrence (decompensation or cirrhosis) at 2 yr for LDLT versus DDLT (45% versus 22%) (OR 2.5, 95% CI 1.1–5.7)

Abbreviations: CI, confidence interval; DDLT, deceased donor liver transplant; LDLT, live donor liver transplant; OR, odds ratio; UNOS, United Network of Organ Sharing.

of mycophenolate mofetil on HCV disease severity is uncertain. In a prospective study comparing tacrolimus, mycophenolate mofetil, and prednisone to tacrolimus and prednisone alone, there were no differences in graft loss or rate of HCV recurrence (although protocol biopsies were not performed) [38]. A recent study found that HCV viral loads increased in patients on a stable regime of cyclosporine and low-dose prednisone when they were changed from azathioprine to mycophenolate mofetil [39]. In a third retrospective study of patients who had recurrent HCV infection, tapering of calcineurin inhibitor therapy with the addition of myeophenolate mofetil was associated with less progression of liver disease compared with patients treated with calcineurin inhibitor tapering only [40]. An initial study of antibody induction therapy suggested a negative impact on HCV disease progression [40], but subsequent studies have not confirmed this finding [41,42]. Sirolimus has not been studied sufficiently to draw conclusions.

A trend reported by some authors is the decreasing graft and patient survival rates over time for patients who have HCV [4,43], which contrasts with

Table 3
Immunosuppression and hepatitis C virus recurrence

Drag	Viral replication	Graft hepatitis
Steroids	Increase + + +	Progression
Cyclosporine	Decrease[a] or stable	No effect
Tacrolimus	Unknown	No effect
MMF	Increase or stable	Controversial
OKT3	Unknown	Controversial
ATG	Unknown	Unknown
Anti-IL2	Unknown	Unknown
Combinations (three or four drags)	Increase + + +	Progression

[a] In cell culture systems.
Data from Refs. [39,45].

the increasing survival rates seen for non-HCV indications during the same time period. There are two changes in clinical practice that have been implicated as the cause for this trend in patients with HCV: (1) the use of newer and more potent immunosuppressive agents [5,35,44] and (2) the increasing use of older donors [23,43,46,47].

Interferon treatment and rejection

In contrast to liver transplant recipients without HCV infection, in whom an episode of acute cellular rejection is associated with improved survival, HCV-infected recipients have a 2.4-fold increase in mortality after an episode of acute rejection [48]. The histologic features of early recurrent HCV infection and acute cellular rejection overlap and make the diagnosis of acute cellular rejection in the setting of recurrent HCV disease difficult [49]. Treatment of recurrent HCV with increased antirejection therapy would be predicted to increase the risk of disease progression, so the issue of misdiagnosis is significant. In a retrospective study of 285 liver transplant recipients, HCV infection was associated with an increased risk of early (<6 months after transplant) acute cellular rejection compared with other transplant indications (HR 1.7) [50]. In this same study, 49% of transplant recipients with HCV infection had at least one episode of early acute cellular rejection. In light of the difficulty in distinguishing mild acute rejection and recurrent HCV from recurrent HCV alone and due to the reported associated between treatment of acute rejection and increased risk of HCV disease progression, some experts have recommended that only acute rejection of moderate or severe degree be treated and that corticosteroid boluses and antibody therapy be used judiciously [51].

Because interferon (IFN) has immunomodulatory effects, specifically the upregulation of HLA expression on bile duct epithelia, there has been concern regarding the risk of rejection related to the use of IFN in liver transplant recipients. This risk of acute rejection may be greater, theoretically, if

IFN is used preemptively rather than later post-transplantation because the risk of acute rejection is highest in the first 3 months after transplantation. Controlled studies of preemptive antiviral treatment strategies have reported similar rates of acute rejection between IFN-treated and control groups [52].

In studies using IFN or peginterferon (PEGIFN) plus ribavirin (RBV) to treat recurrent HCV disease, treatment is initiated typically at least 6 months after transplantation. Two recent uncontrolled retrospective studies of IFN (standard and PEGIFN) plus RBV for the treatment of recurrent hepatitis C showed rates of acute cellular rejection of 11% and 30%, respectively [53,54]. These rates are significantly higher than a previous randomized controlled study [55] and multiple other uncontrolled studies that reported acute rejection rates of 0% to 5% [20,56–63]. Possible explanations for this discrepancy are bias from lack of control subjects, the extended half-life of PEGIFN, heterogeneity in immunosuppression from variable regimens, reduced drug levels, or lower doses of RBV. Chronic rejection rates associated with IFN treatment have ranged from 0% to 4% in controlled and uncontrolled studies, with the exception of one early study reporting a chronic rejection in 5 of 14 IFN-treated subjects [64].

Prevention and treatment of recurrent hepatitis C virus infection

To prevent HCV infection after transplantation, therapies must be given prior to or at the time of transplantation. This prophylactic approach has been successful in the prevention of recurrent HBV infection among transplant recipients [65]. Hepatitis B immune globulin (HBIG) combined with nucleoside analogs can effectively prevent recurrent HBV infection in > 90% of patients. A similarly efficacious therapy has not been identified, however, for HCV-infected patients. In the absence of an effective prophylactic therapy, the focus of studies has been the use of IFN (conventional or PEGIFN) with and without RBV to treat transplant patients preemptively (ie, early in the post-transplant period before clinical onset of recurrent HCV) or later when recurrent and progressive histologic disease is apparent. The latter approach has been the mainstay of management to date, but success has been modest at best (Table 4).

The limited tolerability of IFN and RBV is a major impediment in the treatment of HCV infection in the post-transplant setting. Dose reductions are more common in transplant patients receiving antiviral therapy for recurrent hepatitis C than in nontransplant populations. Dose reductions likely contribute to the lower response rates observed. Cytopenias are frequently due to the concurrent use of immunosuppressive agents and alterations in renal function related to calcineurin inhibitor therapy or other post-transplant factors affecting drug pharmacokinetics. The optimal dose of RBV in transplant patients has not been determined. Perhaps more than in any other treatment population, growth factors to manage

Table 4
Preemptive treatment of hepatitis C virus infection in liver transplant recipients

Study	Study type	n	Treatment regimen	Time to Rx (wk)	SVR	Histologic response	Dose reduction or D/C	F/U (mo)	AR (Rx/ no Rx)
Singh, 1998 [73]	RCT	12 treated, 12 control	IFN, 3MU tiw × 6 mo versus no treatment	2	0% in both groups	No difference in severity	50%	29	6/5
Sheiner, 1998 [71]	RCT	35 IFN, 46 no Rx	IFN 3MU tiw × 6 mo versus no treatment	3	17% IFN; 5% no Rx	Fewer with recurrence at 1 and 2 yr in IFN group	28% drug D/C	22	17/23
Mazzaferro, 2001 [74]	UC	36	IFN 3MU tiw + RBV 10 mg/kg/d for 12 mo	3	33%	Normal biopsy in virologic responders	47%	52	0/–
Shergill, 2004 [70]	RCT (two different Rx arms)	44	IFN/PEGIFN alone versus IFN/ PEGIFN + RBV × 12 mo	≤6	9%	NA	85% dose reductions, 37% D/C	18	18/–
Sugawara, 2004 [75]	UC	21 (all LDLT)	IFN 3MU tiw + RBV 400 mg/d increased to IFN 6MU tiw + RBV 600 mg/d × 12 mo	Median 4.3	43%	Lower HAI score in responders than non-responders	62% dose reductions or discontinuation	26	6/–
Chalasani, 2005 [82]	RCT	26 treated, 28 control	PegIFNα2a 180 μg/wk × 12 mo	3	8% (0% in controls)	No difference in severity	31% drug discontinuation	18	3/6

Abbreviations: AR, acute rejection; D/C, discontinuation: F/U, follow-up time; HAI, hepatic activity index; IFN, interferon; LDLT, living donor liver transplant recipient; MU, million units; PEGIFN, pegylated interferon; RBV, ribavirin; RCT, randomized controlled trial; Rx, treatment; SVR, sustained virologic response; UN, uncontrolled trial.

cytopenias and maintain optimal doses of antiviral treatment are likely to be important in maximizing responses to therapy.

Prophylactic therapy

Preclinical and retrospective cohort data suggest that HCV antibodies have neutralizing effects and may attenuate the risk of HCV infection [66,67]. In a retrospective observational study of transplant recipients with HBV and HCV receiving HBIG, the prevalence of recurrent HCV disease after transplantation was lower in those who received HBIG before screening blood donors for HCV compared with those who received HBIG after routine screening of blood donors for antibody to HCV began [66]. These results suggest that the HCV antibodies in HBIG before screening the donors for HCV infection reduced the risk of recurrent disease. In a study of two chimpanzees treated with high-dose hepatitis C immune globulin (HCIG) immediately before and after HCV inoculation, both animals were initially viremic but subsequently had undetectable HCV RNA and had no evidence of biochemical hepatitis [67].

At least three HCV antibody preparations are being studied in prospective clinical trials [68]. A preliminary report of the Canadian HCIG study found no benefit, with HCV RNA detectable in all treated patients post-transplant and no appreciable difference in the level of viremia or histologic disease in patients receiving HCIG prophylaxis versus control subjects [69]. A second study in the United States evaluated 18 patients (six high-dose HCIG, six low-dose HCIG, and six untreated control subjects) with chronic HCV infection undergoing liver transplantation [70]. Treatment began in the anhepatic phase, and a total of 17 infusions were given over 14 weeks. During treatment, alanine aminotransferase (ALT) levels were lower in treated (especially the high-dose group) than untreated patients, suggesting a possible antiinflammatory effect. There were no differences in serum HCV RNA levels between groups; however, a lower (but not significantly reduced) liver HCV RNA level was noted at month 1 post-transplant in the high-dose group compared with control subjects. In these studies, the HCIG product was produced from anti-HCV positive donors. The studies differed in terms of the doses used and schedule of administration; however, in both studies, reinfection occurred in all patients. A third study, using fully human monoclonal HCV antibodies, is underway, and results are expected in 2005. Based on the data available, however, there is no established role for prophylactic antibody therapy in the management of patients with HCV infection undergoing liver transplantation at this time.

Preemptive antiviral therapy

Preemptive therapy refers to initiation of therapy in the early post-transplant period when HCV viral loads are lower than pretransplant levels, and histologic disease is absent or minimal. These characteristics of the early post-transplant period may enhance virologic responses with antiviral therapy, as has been shown in nontransplant patients. Studies have shown that preemptive antiviral therapy can lead to eradication of HCV infection, but tolerability of therapy is a limitation. Patients with high pretransplant Model for End-stage Liver Disease (MELD) and Child-Turcotte-Pugh scores were less suitable for this therapeutic approach [52]. Unlike nontransplant and acutely infected patients, liver transplant recipients are typically on multiple immunosuppressive drugs and prophylactic antimicrobial agents, have variable renal function, and are recovering from a major operative procedure in the setting of advanced liver disease. All these factors may affect candidacy for and tolerability of HCV therapy. In a study of 110 consecutive patients transplanted for chronic hepatitis C at a single center in the United States, only 60% were found to be candidates for IFN and RBV therapy at 8 weeks post-transplant [52]. Reasons for ineligibility included persistent anemia, renal dysfunction, cardiopuimonary complications, active psychiatric or neurologic diseases, and others reflective of a slower postoperative recovery among patients with advanced liver disease pretransplantation.

Clinical trials using preemptive IFN monotherapy, although generally positive, demonstrated a modest benefit, primarily in delaying time to histologic recurrence. A sustained virologic response (SVR) was infrequent, occurring in 0% to 22% [52,71–73]. A recent study of PegIFNα2a monotherapy for 12 months reported a SVR rate of 8% with high rates of withdrawal due to intolerance (31%) [74]. Studies using IFN and RBV suggest combination therapy is more efficacious. An uncontrolled study from Italy of 36 patients (83% genotype Ib) treated with combination standard IFNα-2b 3 million units (MU) thrice weekly and RBV 10 mg/kg/d within 3 weeks after transplantation and continued for 52 weeks, reported a SVR of 33%, and all patients had normal serum ALT levels and histology after completion of therapy [75]. Viral clearance was more frequent in patients with non-1 HCV genotypes (100%) compared with those with genotype 1b (20%). In contrast to the Italian experience, a United States study of preemptive standard IFN or PEGIFNα-2b 3 MU thrice weekly or 1.5 μg/kg/wk, alone or in combination with RBV 600 mg daily increasing to 1.0 to 1.2 g daily, for a total of 48 weeks, showed an SVR in only 9%, with most responders in the combination group. Dose reductions and discontinuations were required in 85% and 37% of patients, respectively. The inability to achieve full-dose therapy may explain the low SVR rate. The differences in applicability and tolerability of preemptive therapy in the Italian and United States studies may reflect the clinical status of the patients in the early post-transplant period. Whether treating HCV disease preemptively results in better long-term outcomes than treatment initiated only when recurrent disease is established has not been evaluated.

Living donor liver graft recipients may be good candidates for preemptive HCV treatment because they are generally less sick pretransplantation than deceased donor recipients. In an uncontrolled study of 21 HCV-positive recipients of LDLT grafts given IFNα-2b and RBV starting 1 month after transplantation, the SVR was 43% and patient survival was 85%. Six patients (29%) were withdrawn from treatment due to intolerance [76].

Antiviral therapy for recurrent hepatitis C virus disease

In the treatment of established recurrent HCV disease, study protocols have generally initiated treatment between 6 to 24 months after transplantation (Table 5). Initiating treatment after recurrent disease is clinically or histologically apparent, rather than as preemptive treatment, has potential advantages that include lower doses of immunosuppressive drugs (which may enhance the response to antiviral therapy), improved clinical status to better tolerate treatment, lower risk of acute rejection, and cost savings because only those with progressive disease are treated. The potential disadvantages of the approach of "wait and treat" if there is progressive histologic disease include a higher viral load and more advanced stage of fibrosis at the time of treatment, which are factors that may reduce the likelihood of achieving a SVR.

Results with IFN or RBV monotherapy have been disappointing. IFN plus RBV achieves superior results compared to those reported with monotherapy [20,55–63], with histologic improvement reported in both responders and non-responders (Table 5). The majority of the studies evaluating combination therapy for recurrent HCV disease are uncontrolled, use variable doses and duration of IFN and RBV therapy, and are of a sample size too limited to perform multivariate analyses to identify predictors of response. The doses of IFN used in these studies ranged from 1.5 to 5 MU thrice weekly, and the doses of RBV used ranged from 400 to 1200 mg daily; in most studies, the duration of therapy was 48 weeks. End-of-treatment biochemical and virologic responses ranged from 25% to 100% and 9% to 64%, respectively. There was also a wide range of reported SVR rates (assessed at 6 months after completion of therapy) ranging from 5% to 45%. Adverse events during combination treatment are common with withdrawal of treatment, which is required in up to 50% of patients. Anemia, leukopenia, and thrombocytopenia are the most common reasons cited for treatment discontinuation and dose reduction. The SVR rates using PEGIFN plus RBV are typically higher than with standard IFN plus RBV, ranging from 26% to 37.5%. Despite titrated regimens using low initial doses of PEGIFN and RBV, dose reductions and discontinuations are frequently required.

The optimal duration of treatment for recurrent HCV disease is unknown. In immunosuppressed liver transplant recipients, longer treatment periods may be necessary to enhance the SVR. In nontransplant patients who have HCV infection who fail to clear HCV after combination IFN and RBV therapy, maintenance IFN therapy may be beneficial in preventing disease progression and complications of cirrhosis. Although several ongoing clinical trials (HALT-C, EPIC, and CO-PILOT) are investigating this treatment strategy, maintenance therapy has not been evaluated fully as a means of preventing disease progression in liver transplant recipients.

The cost-effectiveness of antiviral therapy for HCV disease in liver transplant recipients has been examined in only one study. Using a Markov-based decision analytic model to simulate costs and health outcomes, treatment of recurrent HCV infection with antiviral therapy (IFN and RBV) was found to be cost effective. Treatment of 100 men, 55 years of age, with recurrent hepatitis C prevented 29 cases of cirrhosis, prevented seven deaths, and had an incremental cost effectiveness ratio of $29,100 per year of life saved [77].

Retransplantation for recurrent hepatitis C virus

The only definitive treatment for patients with advanced recurrent HCV-related liver disease is a repeat liver transplant. Over the next decade, the number of patients with recurrent hepatitis C seeking retransplantation is expected to increase severalfold [78]. In the United States, 8% to 9% of transplants performed are retransplants, with recurrent HCV infection accounting for approximately 40%. Compared with primary transplantation, retransplantation for all indications is associated with longer hospital stays, 40% greater cost, and a 10% to 20% reduction in survival [8]. Outcomes of retransplantation for recurrent HCV disease are reported to be interior to results of retransplantation for other indications. In a large study of over 10,000 patients in the UNOS database, anti-HCV–positive retransplant recipients had reduced survival compared with anti-HCV–negative retransplant recipients, with 5-year survival rates of 54% and 61%, respectively [79]. Studies specifically evaluating retransplantation for recurrent HCV disease (not just HCV-positive status) are smaller and from single centers but show a similar picture. Predictors of poor outcome after retransplantation included recipient age over 50 years, serum creatinine >2.0 mg/dL, serum bilirubin >10 mg/dL, and poor physical condition [80,81]. In general, outcomes are predicted to be best if retransplantation occurs before the onset of liver decompensation or significant renal dysfunction. In a study modeling outcomes of retransplantation, the optimal graft allocation utility function, defined as the product of outcome (predicted post-transplantation survival) and urgency (MELD score), occurred at lower MELD scores for HCV (MELD = 21) compared with non-HCV (MELD = 24) patients [82]. Additionally, those with a longer period of time from first to second transplant seem to have a better outcome [81]. Retransplantation for recurrent HCV disease remains a controversial issue. Most transplant programs use a selective approach, choosing HCV-infected patients with favorable clinical characteristics for retransplantation. Some have advocated that organ allocation

Table 5
Treatment of established recurrent hepatitis C virus disease in liver transplant recipients[a]

Study	Study design	Treatment	n	Average duration time LT to Rx (mo)	W/D N (%)	EOTR N (%)	SVR N (%)	F/U (mo)	AR (Rx/ no Rx)	CR (Rx/ no Rx)
IFN and RBV										
Firpi, 2002 [20]	UC	IFN 3 MU tiw + RBV 800–1000 mg/d × 48 wk	54	31	7 (13)	21 (38)	16 (30)	18	3/–	1/–
Shakil, 2002 [61]	UC	IFN 3 MU tiw + RBV 800 mg/d × 48 wk	38	23	16 (42)	5 (13)	2 (5)	18+	0/–	0/–
Lavezzo, 2002 [62]	UC	IFN 3 MU tiw + RBV 800 mg/kg								
		× 6 mo	27	9	2 (4)	9 (33)	6 (22)	18	1/–	0/–
		× 12 m	30			7 (30)	5 (17)			
Menon, 2002 [63]	UC	IFN 3 MU tiw + RBV 800–100 mg/d × ≥ 12 mo	26	15	13 (50)	9 (35)	6 (23)		0/–	0/–
Bizollon, 2003 [56]	UC	IFN 3 MU tiw + RBV 1000 mg/d × 6 mo then RBV 600–800 mg/d alone × 12 mo	54	13	6 (11)		14 (26)	54	0/–	0/–
Samuel, 2003 [55][b]	RCT	IFN 3 MU tiw + RBV 1000–1200 mg/d × 48 wk	54 (28 treated)	54	12 (43)	9 (32)	6 (21)	18	0/0	1/0
Chalasani, 2005 [74][b]	RCT	PegIFN2a 180 μg/wk × 48 wk	67 (34 untreated)	25	10 (30)	4 (15)[c]	3 (12)[c]	18	4/0	NA
Castells, 2005 [83]	CT	PegIFN2b 1.5 μg/kg/wk + RBV 400–800 mg/d × 48 wk	48 (24 untreated)	3.8	3 (13)	15 (63)[c]	8 (35)[c]	18	1/2	NA

Giostra, 2004 [57]	UC	RBV 10 mg/kg × 12 wk then IFN 3 MU tiw + RBV 10 mg/kg × 48 wk	31	18	9 (29)	14 (45)	9 (31)	18	0/–	1/–
PEGIFN and RBV										
Abdelmalek, 2004 [58]	UC	IFN 3 MU tiw or PEGIFN α-2b 1.5 μg/kg/wk or PEGIFN 90 α-2a μg/wk plus RBV 600–1000 mg/d × 48 wk	90	NA	NA	NA	28 (31)	36	0/–	2/–
Stravitz, 2004 [53]	UC	IFN 3 MU tiw or PEGIFN 1.0 μg/kg/wk RBV 1000 mg/d × 48 wk	23	42	NA	11 (48)	8 (35)	33	7/–	1/–
Saab, 2004 [54]	UC	IFN or PEGIFN and RIB Doses NA	44	42	23 (52)	NA	3 (7)	NA	5/–	0/–
Mukherjee, 2003 [59]	UC	PEGIFN α-2b 1.5 μg/kg/wk × RBV 800/d × 48 wk	39	20	17 (44)	15 (39)	12 (31)	18	NA	NA
Dumortier, 2004 [60]	UC	PEGIFN α-2b 1.0 μg/kg/wk + RBV 1000 mg/d × 48 wk	20	28	4 (20)	11 (55)	9 (45)	18	0/–	0/–

Abbreviations: AR, acute rejection; CR, chronic rejection; CT, controlled trail; F/U, follow-up time; IFN, interferon; MU, million units; N, number; NA, not available; PEGIFN, pegylated interferon; RBV, ribavirin; RCT, randomized controlled trail; UC, uncontrolled trail.

[a] Limited to studies with ≥20 patients.

[b] Only randomized study with untreated control group.

[c] 0 in untreated group.

for retransplantation for HCV and non-HCV etiologies include outcome measures, such as predicted survival after retransplantation, rather than solely wait-list mortality (eg, MELD score) [51,82].

Summary

Recurrent HCV infection is universal in liver transplant recipients who are viremic pretransplant. The rate of histologic disease progression after transplantation is more rapid, and the risk of cirrhosis by 5 to 10 years is about 30%. Several donor, recipient, and viral factors have been associated with worse post-transplant outcomes in recipients with recurrent hepatitis C. Whether or not HCV-infected recipients of live donor grafts have worse outcomes compared with deceased donor graft recipients is controversial. To maximize the long-term survival of recipients with HCV infection, eradication of infection is the ultimate goal. Treatment of recurrent HCV after liver transplantation can be undertaken at several different time points: (1) prophylactically, at the time of transplantation; (2) preemptively, in the early post-transplant period; and (3) after established recurrent histologic disease is present. Prophylactic therapy for HCV infection has no established role at present, but studies are ongoing. Preemptive therapy using IFN and RBV has resulted in variable SVR rates (9%–43%) and is generally poorly tolerated, especially if the patient has advanced liver disease pretransplantation. Treatment of established recurrent HCV disease with combination PEGIFN and RBV is associated with a SVR in about 30% to 35% of patients overall but is limited by high rates of dose reduction or drug discontinuation. In conclusion, successful HCV eradication in the post-transplant setting is difficult with current treatment options, but it is possible. Determination of the optimal doses of antiviral drugs in transplant patients and improvements in drug tolerability may be important first steps in achieving enhanced response rates. There is a need for new drugs in this population that have greater efficacy and a better safety profile.

References

[1] United Network for Organ Sharing. Available at: www.unos.org. Accessed January 11, 2005.
[2] Armstrong G, Alter M, McQuillan G, et al. The past incidence of hepatitis C virus infection: implications for the future burden of chronic liver disease in the United States. Hepatology 2000;31:777–82.
[3] El-Serag HB. Hepatocellular carcinoma and hepatitis C in the United States. Hepatology 2002;36:S74–83.
[4] Forman LM, Lewis JD, Berlin JA, et al. The association between hepatitis C infection and survival after orthotopic liver transplantation. Gastroenterology 2002;122:889–96.
[5] Berenguer M, Ferrell L, Watson J, et al. HCV-related fibrosis progression following liver transplantation: increase in recent years. J Hepatol 2000;32:673–84.

[6] Sanchez-Fueyo A, Restrepo JC, Quinto L, et al. Impact of the recurrence of hepatitis C virus infection after liver transplantation on the long-term viability of the graft. Transplantation 2002;73:56–63.
[7] Gane E, Portmann B, Naoumov N, et al. Long-term outcome of hepatitis C infection after liver transplantation. N Engl J Med 1996;334:815–20.
[8] Biggins S, Terrault N. Should HCV-related cirrhosis be a contraindication for retransplantation? Liver Transpl 2003;9:236–8.
[9] Everson G. Treatment of patients with hepatitis C virus on the waiting list. Liver Transpl 2003;9:S90–4.
[10] Garcia-Retortillo M, Forns X, Feliu A, et al. Hepatitis C virus kinetics during and immediately after liver transplantation. Hepatology 2002;35:680–7.
[11] Fukumoto T, Berg T, Ku Y, et al. Viral dynamics of hepatitis C early after orthotopic liver transplantation: evidence for rapid turnover of serum virions. Hepatology 1996;24:1351–4.
[12] Chazouilleres O, Kim M, Combs C, et al. Quantitation of hepatitis C vims RNA in liver transplant recipients. Gastroenterology 1994;106:994–9.
[13] Sreekumar R, Gonzalez-Koch A, Maor-Kendler Y, et al. Early identification of recipients with progressive histologic recurrence of hepatitis C after liver transplantation. Hepatology 2000;32:1125–30.
[14] Charlton M, Seaberg E, Wiesner R, et al. Predictors of patient and graft survival following liver transplantation for hepatitis C. Hepatology 1998;28:823–30.
[15] Zhou S, Terrault N, Ferrell L, et al. Severity of liver disease in liver transplantation recipients with hepatitis C virus infection: relationship to genotype and level of viremia. Hepatology 1996;24:1041–6.
[16] Crespo J, Carte B, Lozano JL, et al. Hepatitis C virus recurrence after liver transplantation: relationship to anti-HCV core IgM, genotype, and level of viremia. Am J Gastroentero 1997; 92:1458–62.
[17] Gane E, Naoumov N, Qian K, et al. A longitudinal analysis of hepatitis C virus replication following liver transplantation. Gastroenferology 1996;110:167–77.
[18] Taga S, Washington M, Terrault N, et al. Cholestatic hepatitis C in liver allografts. Liver Transpl Surg 1998;4:304–10.
[19] Doughty A, Spencer J, Cossart Y, et al. Cholestatic hepatitis after liver transplantation is associated with persistently high serum hepatitis C virus RNA levels. Liver Transplant Surg 1998;4:15–21.
[20] Firpi R, Abdelmalek M, Soldevila-Pico C, et al. Combination of interferon alfa-2b and ribavirin in liver transplant recipients with histological recurrent hepatitis C. Liver Transpl 2002; 8:1000–6.
[21] Gopal D, Rosen H. Duration of antiviral therapy for cholestatic HCV recurrence may need to be indefinite. Liver Transpl 2003;9:348–53.
[22] Feray C, Caccamo L, Alexander GJ, et al. European collaborative study on factors influencing outcome after liver transplantation for hepatitis C. European Concerted Action on Viral Hepatitis (EUROHEP) Group. Gastroenterology 1999;17:619–25.
[23] Neumann U, Berg T, Bahra M, et al. Fibrosis progression after liver transplantation in patients with recurrent hepatitis C. J Hepatol 2004;41:830–6.
[24] Prieto M, Berenguer M, Rayon J, et al. High incidence of allograft cirrhosis in hepatitis C virus genotype 1b infection following transplantation: relationship with rejection episodes. Hepatoiogy 1999;29:250–6.
[25] Berenguer M, Prieto M, Rayon JM, et al. Natural history of clinically compensated hepatitis C virus-related graft cirrhosis after liver transplantation. Hepatology 2000;32:852–8.
[26] Guido M, Fagiuoli S, Tessari G, et al. Histology predicts cirrhotic evolution of post transplant hepatitis C. Gut 2002;50:697–700.
[27] Thuluvath P, Yoo H. Graft and patient survival after adult live donor liver transplantation compared to a matched cohort who received a deceased donor transplantation. Liver Transpl 2004;10:1263–8.

[28] Russo M, Galanko J, Beavers K, et al. Patient and graft survival in hepatitis C recipients after adult living donor liver transplantation in the United States. Liver Transpl 2004;10: 340–6.
[29] Bozorgzadeh A, Jain A, Ryan C, et al. Impact of hepatitis C viral infection in primary cadaveric liver allograft versus primary living-donor allograft in 100 consecutive liver transplant recipients receiving tacrolimus. Transplantation 2004;77:1066–70.
[30] Gaglio P, Malireddy S, Levitt B, et al. Increased risk of cholestatic hepatitis C in recipients of grafts from living versus cadaveric liver donors. Liver Transpl 2003;9:1028–35.
[31] Shiftman M, Stravitz R, Contos M, et al. Histologic recurrence of chronic hepatitis C virus in patients after living donor and deceased donor liver transplantation. Liver Transpl 2004;10: 1248–55.
[32] Garcia-Retortillo M, Forns X, Llovet J, et al. Hepatitis C recurrence is more severe after living donor compared to cadaveric liver transplantation. Hepatology 2004;40:699–707.
[33] Neumann U, Berg T, Bahra M, et al. Long-term outcome of liver transplants for chronic hepatitis C: a 10-year follow-up. Transplantation 2004;77:226–31.
[34] Eason J, Loss G, Blazek J, et al. Steroid-free liver transplantation using rabbit antithymocyte globulin induction: results of a prospective randomized trial. Liver Transpl 2001;7:693–7.
[35] Papatheodoridis GV, Davies S, Dhillon AP, et al. The role of different immunosuppression in the long-term histological outcome of HCV reinfection after liver transplantation for HCV cirrhosis. Transplantation 2001;72:412–8.
[36] Ghobrial RM, Farmer DG, Baquerizo A, et al. Orthotopic liver transplantation for hepatitis C: outcome, effect of immunosuppression, and causes of retransplantation during an 8-year single-center experience. Ann Surg 1999;229:824–31.
[37] Mueller AR, Platz K, Wiilimski C, et al. Influence of immunosuppression on patient survival after liver transplantation for hepatitis C. Transplant Proc 2001;33:1347–9.
[38] Jain A, Kashyap R, Demetns AJ, et al. A prospective randomized trial of mycophenolate mofetil in liver transplant recipients with hepatitis C. Liver Transpl 2002;8:40–6.
[39] Zekry A, Gleeson M, Guney S, et al. A prospective cross-over study comparing the effect of mycophenolate versus azathioprine on allograft function and viral load in liver transplant recipients with recurrent chronic HCV infection. Liver Transpl 2004;10:52–7.
[40] Bahra M, Neumann U, Jacob D, et al. MMF and calcineurin taper in recurrent hepatitis C after liver transplantation: impact on histological course. Am J Transplant 2005;5: 406–11.
[41] Neuhaus P, Clavien P, Kittur D, et al. Improved treatment response with basiliximab immunoprophylaxis after liver transplantation: results from a double-blind randomized placebo-controlled trial. Liver Transpl 2002;8:132–42.
[42] Calmus Y, Scheele J, Gonzalez-Pinto I, et al. Immunoprophylaxis with basiliximab, a chimeric anti-interleukin-2 receptor monoclonal antibody, in combination with azathioprine-containing triple therapy in liver transplant recipients. Liver Transpl 2002;8:123–31.
[43] Burak KW, Kremers WK, Batts KP, et al. Impact of cytomegalovirus infection, year of transplantation, and donor age on outcomes after fiver transplantation for hepatitis C. Liver Transpl 2002;8:362–9.
[44] McCaughan G, Zekry A. Impact of immunosuppression on immunopathogenesis of liver damage in hepatitis C virus-infected recipients following liver transplantation. Liver Transpl 2003;9:S21–7.
[45] Nelson DR, Soldevila-Pico C, Reed A, et al. Anti-interleukin-2 receptor therapy in combination with mycophenolate mofetil is associated with more severe hepatitis C recurrence after liver transplantation. Liver Transpl 2001;7:1064–70.
[46] Berenguer M, Prieto M, San Juan F, et al. Contribution of donor age to the recent decrease in patient survival among HCV-infected liver transplant recipients. Hepatology 2002;36: 202–10.
[47] Wali M, Harrison RF, Gow PJ, et al. Advancing donor liver age and rapid fibrosis progression following transplantation for hepatitis C. Gut 2002;51:248–52.

[48] Charlton M, Seaberg E. Impact of immunosuppression and acute rejection on recurrence of hepatitis C: results of the National Institute of Diabetes and Digestive and Kidney Diseases Liver Transplantation Database. Liver Transpl Surg 1999;5:S107–14.
[49] Regev A, Molina E, Maura R, et al. Reliability of histopathologic assessment for the differentiation of recurrent hepatitis C from acute rejection after liver transplantation. Liver Transpl 2004;10:1233–9.
[50] McTaggart R, Terrault N, Vardanian A, et al. Hepatitis C etiology of liver disease is strongly associated with early acute rejection following liver transplantation. Liver Transpl 2004;10: 975–85.
[51] Wiesner R, Sorrell M, Villamil F. International Liver Transplantation Society Expert Panel. Report of the first International Liver Transplantation Society expert panel consensus conference on liver transplantation and hepatitis C. Liver Transpl 2003;9:S1–9.
[52] Shergill A, Khalili M, Bellinger K, et al. Applicability, tolerability and efficacy of preemptive antiviral therapy in hepatitis C infected patients undergoing liver transplantation. Am J Transplant 2005;5:118–24.
[53] Stravitz R, Shiftman M, Sanyal A, et al. Effects of interferon treatment on liver histology and allograft rejection in patients with recurrent hepatitis C following liver transplantation. Liver Transpl 2004;10:850–8.
[54] Saab S, Kalmaz D, Gajjar N, et al. Outcomes of acute rejection after interferon therapy in liver transplant recipients. Liver Transpl 2004;10:859–67.
[55] Samuel D, Bizollon T, Feray C, et al. Interferon-alpha 2b plus ribavirin in patients with chronic hepatitis C after liver transplantation: a randomized study. Gastroenterology 2003;124:642–50.
[56] Bizollon T, Ahmed S, Radenne S, et al. Long term histological improvement and clearance of intrahepatic hepatitis C virus RNA following sustained response to interferon-ribavirin combination therapy in liver transplanted patients with hepatitis C virus recurrence. Gut 2003;52:283–7.
[57] Giostra E, Kullak-Ublick G, Keller W, et al. Ribavirin/interferon-alpha sequential treatment of recurrent hepatitis C after liver transplantation. Transpl Int 2004;17:169–76.
[58] Abdelmalek M, Firpi R, Soldevila-Pico C, et al. Sustained viral response to interferon and ribavirin in liver transplant recipients with recurrent hepatitis C. Liver Transpl 2004;10: 199–207.
[59] Mukherjee S, Rogge J, Weaver L, et al. Pilot study of pegylated interferon alfa-2b and ribavirin for recurrent hepatitis C after liver transplantation. Transplant Proc 2003;35:3042–4.
[60] Dumortier J, Scoazec J, Chevallier P, et al. Treatment of recurrent hepatitis C after liver transplantation: a pilot study of peginterferon alfa-2b and ribavirin combination. J Hepatol 2004;40:669–74.
[61] Shakil AO, McGuire B, Crippin J, et al. A pilot study of interferon alfa and ribavirin combination in liver transplant recipients with recurrent hepatitis C. Hepatology 2002;36: 1253–8.
[62] Lavezzo B, Franchello A, Smedile A, et al. Treatment of recurrent hepatitis C in liver transplants: efficacy of a six versus a twelve month course of interferon alfa 2b with ribavirin. J Hepatol 2002;37:247–52.
[63] Narayanan Menon KV, Poterucha JJ, El-Amin OM, et al. Treatment of posttransplantation recurrence of hepatitis C with interferon and ribavirin: lessons on tolerability and efficacy. Liver Transpl 2002;8:623–9.
[64] Feray C, Samuel D, Gigou M, et al. An open trial of interferon alfa recombinant for hepatitis C after liver transplantation: antiviral effects and risk of rejection. Hepatology 1995;22: 1084–9.
[65] Terrault N. Hepatitis B and liver transplantation. Semin Gastrointest Dis 2000;11:96–114.
[66] Feray C, Gigou M, Samuel D, et al. Incidence of hepatitis C in patients receiving different preparations of hepatitis B immunoglobulins after liver transplantation. Ann Intern Med 1998;128:810–6.

[67] Krawczynski K, Alter M, Tankersley D, et al. Effect of immune globulin on the prevention of experimental hepatitis C virus infection. J Infect Dis 1996;173:822–8.
[68] Terrault N. Prophylactic and preemptive therapies for hepatitis C virus-infected patients undergoing liver transplantation. Liver Transpl 2003;9:S95–100.
[69] Willems B, Marotta P, Greig PD, et al. Anti-HCV immunoglobulins for the prevention of graft infection in HCV-related liver transplantation. J Hepatol 2002;36:S96A.
[70] Davis GL, Nelson DR, Terrault NA, et al. A randomized, open-label study to evaluate the safety and pharmacokinetics of human hepatitis C immune globulin (Civacir) in liver transplant recipients. Liver Transpl 2005;11:941–9.
[71] Sheiner P, Boros P, Klion F, et al. The efficacy of prophylactic interferon alfa-2b in preventing recurrent hepatitis C after liver transplantation. Hepatology 1998;28:831–8.
[72] Reddy K, Wippler D, Zervos X, et al. Recurrent HCV infection following liver transplantation: the role of early post transplant interferon treatment. Hepatology 1996;24:295A.
[73] Singh N, Gayowski T, Wannstedt CF, et al. Interferon-alpha for prophylaxis of recurrent viral hepatitis C in liver transplant recipients: a prospective, randomized, controlled trial. Transplantation 1998;65:82–6.
[74] Chalasani N, Manzarbeitia C, Ferenci P, et al. Peginterferon alfa-2a for hepatitis C after liver transplantation: two randomized, controlled trials. Hepatology 2005 Feb;41:289–98.
[75] Mazzaferro V, Tagger A, Schiavo M, et al. Prevention of recurrent hepatitis C after liver transplantation with early interferon and ribavirin treatment. Transplant Proc 2001;33: 1355–7.
[76] Sugawara Y, Makuuchi M, Matsui Y, et al. Preemptive therapy for hepatitis C virus after living-donor liver transplantation. Transplantation 2004;78:1308–11.
[77] Saab S, Ly D, Han SB, et al. Is it cost-effective to treat recurrent hepatitis C injection in OLT patients. Liver Transpl 2002;8:449–57.
[78] Wall W, Khakhar A. Retransplantation for recurrent hepatitis C: the argument against. Liver Transpl 2003;9:S73–8.
[79] Rosen HR, Madden JP, Martin P. A model to predict survival following liver retransplantation. Hepatology 1999;29:365–70.
[80] Neff G, O'Brien C, Nery J, et al. Factors that identify survival after liver retransplantation for allograft failure caused by recurrent hepatitis C infection. Liver Transpl 2004;10: 1497–503.
[81] Rosen H. Validation and refinement of survival models for liver retransplantation. Hepatology 2003;38:460–9.
[82] Burton JJ, Sonnenberg A, Rosen H. Retransplantation for recurrent hepatitis C in the MELD era: maximizing utility. Liver Transpl 2004;10(Suppl 2):S59–64.
[83] Castells L, Vargas V, Allende H, et al. Combined treatment with pegylated interferon (alpha-2b) and ribavirin in the acute phase of hepatitis C virus recurrence after liver transplantation. J Hepatol 2005;43:53–9.

ELSEVIER
SAUNDERS

Infect Dis Clin N Am
20 (2006) 175–178

INFECTIOUS
DISEASE CLINICS
OF NORTH AMERICA

Index

Note: Page numbers of article titles are in **boldface** type.

0891-5520/06/$ - see front matter
doi:10.1016/S0891-5520(06)00028-6 *id.theclinics.com*